# THE NHS –
# UNDER NEW MANAGEMENT

# THE NHS –
# UNDER NEW MANAGEMENT

Philip Strong
and
Jane Robinson

Open University Press
Milton Keynes · Philadelphia

Open University Press
Celtic Court
22 Ballmoor
Buckingham
MK18 1XW

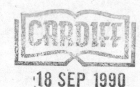

and
1900 Frost Road, Suite 101
Bristol, PA 19007, USA

First published 1990

Copyright © P. Strong and J. Robinson 1990

*British Library Cataloguing in Publication Data*

Strong, Philip
    The N.H.S. – under new management.
    1. Great Britain. National Health Services. Management
    I. Title   II. Robinson, Jane
    362.1068

    ISBN  0  335  09296  9
          0  335  09295  0  pbk

*Library of Congress Cataloging-in-Publication Data*

Strong, Philip, 1945–
    The NHS – under new management/Philip Strong, Jane Robinson.
       p.   cm.
    ISBN 0-335-09296-9.     ISBN 0-335-09295-0 (pbk.)
    1. National Health Service (Great Britain) – Management. 2. Health
services administration – Great Britain.   I. Robinson, Jane, 1935–
II. Title.
    RA241.S87 1990
    362.1′0941 – dc20                                    89-77104 CIP

Typeset by Inforum Typesetting, Portsmouth
Printed in Great Britain by St Edmundsbury Press Ltd
Bury St Edmunds, Suffolk

# Contents

One may say that the Industrial Revolution has finally caught up with medicine and that the medical practitioner is being brought into the 'factory' . . . where he is being subjected to the necessary 'labour disciplines'.

George Rosen, American historian of medicine, cited in 1972[1]

If there's a hole in a' your coats
I rede you tent it:
A chield's amang you takin' notes
And faith he'll prent it.

Robert Burns, 1789[2]

# Foreword

Between 1837 and 1841, so it appears, George Whistler introduced the first modern management system into business.[1] Whistler was the Superintendent of the Western Railroad of Boston, Massachusetts (and the father of the painter, James Whistler). He placed himself and a small headquarters staff at the hub of the organization. The rest he separated into three operating divisions: engineering, transport and maintenance. The new principle he introduced to the business was that of continuous accountability: detailed management was delegated to the divisions but it was simultaneously made subject to constant, systematic monitoring. Each division had to report on a daily, weekly and monthly basis, supplying financial and performance data to the central office staff for their regular appraisal and (where necessary) intervention.

Whistler's main inspiration for this system had come from new methods of assessment and management in the world of higher education, from Sylvanus Thayer at the West Point Military Academy (where Whistler had been cadet staff sergeant major) and from the Ecole Polytechnique in Paris where Thayer himself had been trained. But, if a key part of the origins of modern management lay in the groves of academe, its impact on the world was long confined almost exclusively to business. Indeed, it was not until 1984, almost one hundred and fifty years after George Whistler started work at the Western Railroad, that the modern version of the system arrived in British health care. This book is a case-study of that arrival, of the beginnings of a huge change in health sector management. It focuses, above all, on the new managers themselves: on their diagnosis of the problems that face British health care, on their analysis of both the old and the new methods of working, on their vision of the future.

If one part of the book tries to describe, the other tries to assess. The application of general management – as the system is now currently known – presents a fundamental challenge, not just to the way public health services have been organized since 1948 but also to the way most Britons have thought about these matters for many years. Britons have grown used to seeing health care as quite distinct from the world of business, as a separate, perhaps higher, realm with its own personnel, principles, motives and methods of organization. This doctrine of health care exceptionalism is now confronted head on by the universal claims made by the theory that has come to dominate most modern businesses and business schools.

General management rests on the argument that there are profound similarities between all large organizations, regardless of their particular activities, workforce or clientele. Anywhere and everywhere you look, so it is claimed, much the same practical problems occur, problems which are most effectively solved by a common set of managerial methods. Every effective business or service organization needs firm leadership, the systematic specification of goals, the detailed measurement of individual and group performance and a battery of rewards and punishments. Such methods must be used in a single line of command which stretches from the very top to the bottom of the organization. Every tier must have its leader who monitors, integrates and controls all those who work within that tier and every such leader must be directly responsible to the leader of the tier above. Without such methods, so it is argued, there is an inexorable tendency for the workforce to wander off and do their own thing. However technically skilled or highly motivated, people tend to end up doing work that is expensive, sloppy, ill coordinated and not quite what the customer actually needs.

Until 1984, however, the NHS was organized on quite a different principle. Like general managers, the men and women who created the NHS believed in very firm central control. The highest of all management tiers – that of ministers and civil servants – had a very tight grip. But, in certain key respects, that grip extended no further than Whitehall. The tiers below were a different story. Ministers ruled the health service – with its workforce of nearly a million – with the very thinnest of administrative veneers. Such economy was made possible, not through monitoring the work of individual employees, but through a delegation of power to the most crucial health service trade – the doctors.

The method was simple. Doctors were given support services, placed under a few tight financial and administrative constraints, then left to get on with the service in the ways each practitioner thought most fit. Doctors had no boss and their individual performance went unmonitored. At the frontline medicine was merely administered, not managed. Despite such absences, the NHS was a success. The method might not square with the theory of general management but, judged by international standards, it worked well enough. The NHS produced medical care of high technical quality, delivered it in a reasonably egalitarian fashion and did so at remarkably little cost to the taxpayer.

So, if it wasn't bust, why fix it? Various guesses may be made as to the motives of the Thatcher administration, some less, some more creditable. To some defenders of the old NHS, the system, far from needing reform, has been a shining model to the rest of the world. Of course the service has had problems, but these have been minor when compared with its virtues. What it needed, if anything, was more money, not more management. According to this account, the new doctrines introduced in 1984 were merely an ideological mask to cover the dubious aspirations of businessmen, right-wing politicians and ambitious health service administrators.

Such an account is not wholly implausible, but there would seem to have been many other motives, too. Health care has always been massively shaped by the rest of the economy and as the industrial revolution continues to evolve, so too does the health care system. The old NHS rested on a deal made forty years ago and much has changed since that time. Computer technology has introduced new micro-management techniques. The push to control doctors is not a British but a worldwide phenomenon that affects every Western industrialized country. And in every sector of the economy, both public and private, most countries are currently employing much more systematic management in the twin search for productivity and quality.

None the less, what may sometimes look inevitable from the perspective of hindsight is a lot less so when viewed in close up. Though every Western industrialized society now has an elaborate welfare state, their forms still differ markedly and some seem to work better than others. Introducing radical change into a system that has done quite well up until now is a risky business. Some sort of evaluation is needed. Of course, in one crucial respect any evaluation comes too late. Whatever the rights and wrongs of the case, there is no going back on general management. No politician would willingly give up the power it offers over doctors. But there are still many other choices to be made. General management has only just begun to be applied to health care and it may develop in many different ways.

Indeed, in early 1989, as we started to revise the earlier report on which this book is based,[2] a government White Paper promised yet further major transformation of the NHS;[3] a transformation which is still being fought, over six months later. Whatever the immediate outcome, these battles will continue. The revolution that general management promises in health care is still in its very earliest stages. There is still much to learn and many complex decisions to be made.

How, then, can we best choose between the proposals on offer? In academic terms, there are many different ways of approaching the problem: systematic analysis of the organizational and management literature on other sectors; historical and political inquiry into the origins, trajectory and consequences of health service reorganization; epidemiological and economic research into the costs and effectiveness of different methods of running health care; international comparisons between one health system and another. All these are needed. So too is ethnography, of which this book is an example.

A variety of ethnographic studies of the Griffiths reorganization have been undertaken, for the technique is now used by many different disciplines and in many different ways.[4] The method stems originally from anthropology but has close parallels with some of the methods used by social historians. Both sorts of research aim to study thought and belief and the way these relate to human action. How can this be done? Some thoughts and beliefs remain unsaid, some are deliberately concealed, but many are spoken or written down. This ethnography of the new mode of managing the NHS sets out to capture speech rather than the written word. To do this, we sat in on internal health service management meetings; we attended conferences at which the doctrines of the new management were explained; but, above all, we conducted lengthy informal interviews with people directly involved in health service management – with doctors, nurses, general managers, directors of finance and personnel and with the chairmen of health authorities (as all those who sit in the chair are officially known, regardless of their gender).

The NHS is a vast organization and ethnography is an intensive method. Although we wished to portray the whole, we were forced to be selective. Though data on the new vision were gathered from managers at many different levels, we focused our main efforts on the middle structure of management, on the district tier, located halfway between the ward sister and the Secretary of State. Since districts were both complex and widely varying, a further selection was necessary. Though fragments of data were gathered from many different districts, the main part of our study focused on seven in more detail.

So this is a middling view of the new NHS management: one which looks across to other districts, which peers down at individual hospitals, clinicians and cleaners and which gazes up to the tiers above – to region and, beyond that, to Whitehall. As such, the view also reflects districts' own priorities at this time. Local as well as national politicians are important. Hospitals get a lot more room than community care. GPs are hardly considered, since they are outside districts' control.

But if the view is dictated partly by districts' priorities, it is also shaped by ours. Though our study covers many different aspects of NHS management, it had its origins solely in nurse management. Nursing is typically neglected in most health service discussions. Doctors – and now managers – get all the attention. But, although the modern NHS cannot be understood without close scrutiny of doctors and general managers, it is foolish to ignore nursing. With nurses comprising one-half of the workforce and costing one-third of the revenue budget, nursing needs careful examination. Our study, then, aims both to contribute to a general understanding of health care and management and to accord nursing the place within that management that its size, cost and importance rightfully deserve.

One last, chronological point on perspective. This study of district managers and their views was conducted at various times between the autumn of 1985 and the summer of 1987. When the study began, the old administration was either buried or waiting for death. But, though general management was now firmly in place, the past was still fresh in everyone's mind, while the new structures had all the vividness that novelty inspires. Indeed, those to whom we listened were all driven by the shock of the new, by the tidal wave of change that had swept over the service, a tide that washed over all NHS managers whether they liked it or not. Some feared it; others found it cleansing and invigorating. Huge efforts were required to swim with the tide. Some were exhilarated and rode it like surfers, others were swept away, never to surface again.

So this is a story about people trying to cope with, understand and implement change. The story has five parts. The first provides some essential background. It summarizes some key issues in health care organization, describes the structure of the NHS – old and new – and considers the methods we have used to study it. The second part considers the frontline staff, the doctors and nurses and their complex relations, both to each other and to managers. The third part outlines the ambitious new model of management which aimed to put the clinical trades on an integrated, monitored and subordinate footing. The fourth part considers the huge variations with which the new managers had to deal – the enormous diversity of local hospitals, populations and politicians. The fifth and final part tries to stand back a little and evaluate both the reforms of 1984 and those proposed in 1989, for that further reorganization plans to build on the foundations that were laid in 1984.

But, before we begin, a few pieces of consumer advice. The NHS is not only the largest organization in Britain, it is also undoubtedly the most complex. So one of our main aims is to convey some sense of the extraordinary intricacy of the NHS; of the innumerable patterns and interconnections that it contains; of the complexity that is, in fact, beyond anyone's full comprehension. Like everyone else, what we can see is only a part of the whole.

A second word of warning. This is a book that can be read in many different ways. Managers (so we hope) may read it to see what their colleagues have to say and to reflect upon their own actions. Students may read it to learn something of health service management. Academics and policy makers may read it to help evaluate the new methods of organization. Sociologists may read it as an example of ethnographic study. Different purposes dictate different uses. Some readers may get most from simply dipping into the quotations, others may prefer to study the whole. Those who are unfamiliar with health care and its management might pay close attention to the first part of the book which gives some background to these matters; others may choose to skip most of this section and proceed straight to the core. The choice, as always, is the reader's.

The same choice applies to the quotations we have used. After the first background chapters, much of the rest of the story is told in managers' own words. Their speech is set inside an analytic framework which we ourselves provide but the evidence for our arguments comes in clusters of quotation – two, three, four, even five quotations may be pulled together to illustrate a point. Some of the quotations are short, others are long and complex. Most stem from interviews or speeches at conferences, others are taken from management meetings. Those who wish to study the main thrust of an argument may focus on just one or two quotations; those who wish to explore its complexities may prefer to read them all.

Two final points on the identity of those to whom we talked. Since almost everyone spoke so frankly, we have omitted most names, invented new ones and changed what identifying details we could. A similar blanket of anonymity has been thrown over districts. This necessary anonymity is increased by our copious use of acronyms. All large organizations use shorthand terms to describe their managerial posts and the NHS is no exception. Most of the time, when citing quotations from our data, we give merely the acronym, not the speaker's full title. A complete guide – including a few of our very own creation – is given in an appendix.

# Acknowledgements

We would like to thank the King Edward's Hospital Fund for its generous financial support to the Nursing Policy Studies Centre at the University of Warwick. That backing gave us the opportunity to do independent research into NHS management. We are also enormously indebted to all those who participated in the research and were so remarkably open and friendly, especially at a time of great individual and organizational stress. We must also thank our many academic colleagues who helped us at key points with topic, theory, method, design and interpretation. A special obligation is owed to John Perrins for a conversation early in 1985 from which the idea of a study of Griffiths emerged; to Meg Stacey for chairing our own management team and keeping us both in line; to Nick Black and Alastair Gray for their many crucial comments on health service matters as the research progressed; to Graham Burchill for his reflections on the new modes of government in the 1980s; to Anne Murcott for her careful reading of the final manuscript and her methodological analysis of what we had actually done; and to the publishers' reviewers for their helpful suggestions. Finally, we must also thank our partners, Anne Murcott (a double duty) and Robbie Robinson, for their patience and support during the lengthy and, at times, stressful conduct of this project.

# List of abbreviations

| | |
|---|---|
| A and E | Accident and emergency |
| ADNS | Assistant director of nursing services |
| BM | Business manager |
| BMA | British Medical Association |
| CAT | Computer-assisted tomography |
| CHC | Community health council |
| CNA | Chief nurse advisor |
| CNO | Chief nursing officer (CANO in Wales) |
| COHSE | Confederation of Health Service Employees |
| DA | District administrator |
| DCh | District chairman |
| DDQ | District director of quality |
| DDR | District director of research |
| DEO | District estates officer |
| DFD | District finance director |
| DGH | District general hospital |
| DGM | District general manager |
| DHA | District health authority |
| DHSS | Department of Health and Social Security |
| DID | District information director |
| DMO | District medical officer |
| DMT | District management team |
| DNE | Director of nurse education |
| DNO | District nursing officer |
| DNS | Director of nursing service |
| DPO (DPD) | District personnel officer/director |
| DR | District research |
| DRG | Diagnostic related groupings |
| EAG | Educational advisory group |
| ENB | English National Board |
| ENT | Ear, nose and throat |
| FPC | Family practitioner committee |

| | |
|---|---|
| GMC | General Medical Council |
| GNC | General Nursing Council |
| GNP | Gross National Product |
| GP | General practitioner |
| HA | Health authority |
| HAA | Hospital activity analysis |
| HQ | Headquarters |
| HSR | Health services researcher |
| IHSM | Institute of Health Service Management |
| INT | Interviewer |
| ITU | Intensive therapy unit |
| JCC | Joint consultative committee |
| MAC | Medical advisory committee |
| MC | Management consultant |
| MH | Mental handicap |
| ML | Management lecturer |
| MOH | Medical officer of health |
| NAHA | National Association of Health Authorities |
| NAO | National Audit Office |
| NCB | National Coal Board |
| NHS | National Health Service |
| NHSBM | National Health Service board member |
| NMPAC(G) | Nursing and midwifery professional advisory committee (group) |
| PAC | Professional advisory committee |
| PI | Performance indicator |
| PSGM | Private sector hospital general manager |
| R and D | Research and development |
| RAWP | Resource Allocation Working Party |
| RCN | Royal College of Nursing |
| RCh | Regional chairman |
| RDP | Regional director of planning |
| RFD | Regional finance director |
| RGM | Regional general manager |
| RHA | Regional health authority |
| RMO | Regional medical officer |
| RNO | Regional nursing officer |
| RPD | Regional personnel director |
| RPO | Regional personnel officer |
| SCM | Specialist in community medicine |
| SDMB | Secretary to the district management board |
| UFD | Unit finance director |
| UGM | Unit general manager |
| UKCC | United Kingdom Central Council for Nursing, Midwifery and Health Visiting |

| | |
|---|---|
| UMT | Unit management team |
| UNO(NO) | Unit nursing officer |
| USGM | American hospital general manager |
| USVPM | American hospital vice president of medicine |
| VFM | Value for money |
| YTS | Youth Training Scheme |

# PART I INTRODUCTION

# 1    Outline and methods

The Royal Lancaster Hotel is a large, ugly, modern building on London's Bayswater Road. Just five minutes' walk from Paddington station and ten minutes' from Marble Arch, it squats directly over the Central line: a convenient, if anonymous, spot for a conference. Throughout 1985 and 1986, senior NHS administrative staff were regular visitors. Chairmen of health authorities, directors of finance and personnel, community physicians, nurse managers, general managers and aspirants to management would sit, several hundred strong, and listen to the prophets of the new order: leading businessmen, pioneering administrators, reforming researchers and members of the new NHS management board. In the heady atmosphere that a day off work can induce, a dream was outlined; a vision that was both organizational and moral. All the gossip over lunch might be of jobs and new appointments, but this was not just another way of structuring the health service, it was also a crusade. The vast, million-strong organization was being remoulded along new and highly radical lines.

'Griffiths', or 'general management', as the crusade was known, was an efficiency drive. (Griffiths was the businessman who had chaired the inquiry in 1983 which led to the reorganization in 1984.)[1] But Griffiths was more than a quest for greater economy. It was also, or so it was hoped, a far better way of running health services; a way in which higher quality care would be delivered from coordinated frontline workers. Down the tatty corridors of the NHS, new and dedicated heroes would stride – the general managers. Inspired by their leadership a new sort of staff would arise. Armed with better information and new techniques from the private sector, much more closely monitored yet working as a team, they would at last take collective pride in their work – and responsibility for it. Something of this vision is captured in the following extract from one such conference. The talk – 'NHS plc' – was given by a district general manager, one of the few to come in from the private sector.

> We've had a start this morning, a very good start indeed [from a leading businessman]. We've got our other stars later this afternoon. I'm the guy who does the warm up after that marvellous lunch! The reason I chose 'NHS plc' as a topic is that, as an ex-management consultant, I went through exactly the same process in thinking about the NHS as I would have done if I was going to look into any company in

order to help it . . . OK, then, let's look at this great organization, the NHS plc. There's a holding company – which is the DHSS and the NHS management board; there are industrial groups – the regions; there are manufacturing companies – the districts; and then there are the factories and the outworkers – the units. Now, that's all very well, but if you're creating a product, you have to have direct and indirect workers. The direct workers are the clinicians, the GPs, the paramedics and the nurses. The indirect workers are finance, personnel, works, the administrators, the clerks and the hotel services side. The important thing . . . to understand is that there is total interdependence between the two. I find it very unfortunate to hear consultants say, 'We're the only important people in the hospital, all the rest are merely here to serve us'. I find this attitude frightening. Everyone has to contribute . . . What we're talking about in Griffiths is not the introduction of *general* management, but the introduction of *proper* management. General managers are being brought in to ensure this . . . They're the catalysts, the people who have to recognize how to control things operationally, to state common objectives – that we're all here to deliver health care . . . I'm very glad to be part of it. If we can pull people in to do it properly, we shall all move forward. That's what I'm here for and that's what you're here for. [Added emphasis]

To understand the message and the fervour, compare another sort of image of the NHS, an image provided, not by managers but by the profession of medicine. If Griffiths meant NHS plc, many doctors saw the NHS rather ✳ differently. [In the conventional medical view, the NHS was a system for servicing individual clinicians. Doctors, not managers, ruled. Indeed, there were no managers. The local health service was merely administered by low-level functionaries on behalf of its leaders, the doctors. Managers were for the business world, but frontline health care was different. Fundamentally dependent on scientific expertise but simultaneously providing the most personal and vital of services, clinical care was a matter for the professions, not for bureaucrats.]Speaking to journalists in 1985, the hospital consultants' spokesman, Paddy Ross, defended the old ways against the new:

The concept of the NHS was to provide an administrative system within which doctors treated patients in the light of their professional judgment. The NHS is just the system that pays the bills and provides the hospitals and all that.[2]

Many occupations have such dreams but what is most striking about this view is its essential truth. This is the way the NHS was organized, in most crucial respects, in the first forty years of its existence. The NHS was a pyramid. Perched high on its apex stood the thirty thousand doctors – consultants a little above the general practitioners. Each had to cope with the grave responsibility of managing disease but each had also been trained in the best of modern scientific medicine. Below them, stretching out in ever vaster numbers towards the base of the pyramid, came the support staff; those who nurtured, and aided the work of each doctor – around a million in total. On one side, stood the subordinate men: engineers, porters, administrators, ambulancemen, groundsmen, accountants, electricians, psychiatric nurses and scientists without medical degrees. On the other side, were the subordinate women: general nurses, cleaners, clerks, social workers, health visitors, midwives, laboratory technicians, the 'professions ancillary to medicine'. But, although the jobs and genders might differ, they were handmaidens all; serving medicine as medicine, in turn, served each patient – or so the old theory went.

## The origins of the study

This book is about the assault on the old ways; about the ending of mere administration and the attempt, after so many decades, to substitute managerial for medical leadership at every tier of the service. But although this is its focus, its origins lie in one-half of the pyramid, among the subordinate women. Though medicine was the chief target of the Griffiths reforms, nursing was the group that most immediately suffered. The power of doctors was too great for an initial assault; too great, indeed, even to get a mention in the 1983 management inquiry. Managers moved slowly and had to cover their tracks. But with nurses it was different. Nursing might be the biggest of the health service trades and the largest single item of health service expenditure, but its influence was weak and its affairs almost unknown outside nursing circles. At a stroke, the 1984 reorganization removed nursing from nursing's own control and placed it firmly under the new general managers.

Although there was relatively little public fuss some stir was created, enough to prompt the Nursing Policy Studies Centre at the University of Warwick to undertake an inquiry of its own. The research was conducted by its two senior staff, the authors of the current book. (Jane Robinson, then the director of the centre, is a health services researcher who has previously worked as both a clinical nurse and a nurse manager. Philip Strong, then the principal research fellow, is a sociologist whose earlier work had concentrated primarily on doctors.) The new study focused initially on the main change that Griffiths created for nurses. The chief officers who had once managed nursing were now demoted to advisory status. While the new general managers might listen to nursing advice, it was they – not nurses – who now ultimately controlled the budget and the workforce. To gain some idea of what had happened and why, and which direction the management of nursing might take in the future, the first months were spent exploring a variety of management settings. On the basis of this preliminary research, it was decided to focus the main part of the research at the district tier of management. Seven widely varying districts were selected for particular study, three of them with a national reputation for innovation in the management of nursing (though data were gathered from a good many other districts).

These districts were studied in two rounds of research. The first started in January 1986 and lasted six months. In this period, most of the senior district managers then in post were interviewed. The second, much more rapid round, came a year later in 1987, when just the district general managers and chief nurse advisors were spoken to. But, though district was the core, it was not the sole part of our study: DHSS, regions, units and professional gatherings also came in for some share of the research. In all, twelve management conferences, seventeen meetings of district health authorities, thirteen meetings of nursing and midwifery professional advisory groups, four meetings of district management boards and two meetings of senior nurse managers were attended. One hundred and forty informal interviews were also conducted, some of which were recorded by hand, others on audiotape (no distinction is made between these in the text that follows). Finally, as the research progressed, eighteen seminars were given to managers of various kinds.

## The study's focus and research philosophy

If the project had its origins in nursing and its management, one part of the study grew rapidly in its scale and its breadth. Elsewhere, the research focused more directly on the problems of chief nurse advisors.[3] In the work reported here, a more global view was taken. Nursing, although vast, was merely one part of the whole and a part that was definitely subordinate. Many of its options and dilemmas could not be properly grasped without paying systematic attention to the rest of the service, to medicine, finance, personnel, administration and the technical problems that face all health care systems.

The management of nursing, therefore, needed a context. A very general study was called for, one which surveyed the whole of Griffiths and not just its impact on the old chief nursing officers. None the less, the CNOs and their successors were a good place to start. CNOs had been part of the district management team for a decade, while the nurses they controlled covered every part of the service. Much might be learnt about the NHS from this perspective, providing it was balanced by the views of the rest of the management team – which is what we set out to do. To this end, the interviews ranged far and wide, while the data these produced were analysed through 'constant comparison' and 'analytic induction' – methods for generating systematic description of a vast range of analytic categories.[4]

This book, then, is not a study of nursing but an analysis of the huge wave of change that swept across NHS management in the years that followed 1984. It deals with the dilemmas and solutions, the experience and opinions, the hopes and the fears, the tactics and strategies, the perspectives and ideologies of the new management class as it struggled in the mid-1980s to make sense of, and to implement, Griffiths.

Because of this, the main theme of this work is fairly abstract. Organizations are complex phenomena. Any institution is built out of the relationships between human beings. Since just two people can have a most intricate relationship, an organization like the NHS – which has nearly a million members – is quite extraordinarily complex. Diagrams and charts which portray its formal structure on a page necessarily fail to capture the whole. To help solve this dilemma, social science makes a fundamental distinction between the formal and informal aspects of organizations, between the official rhetoric and what actually happens. Each, of course, influences the other. The formal sphere shapes informal action; the unofficial sphere, in its turn, is oriented to and may partially modify the official form of things.[5]

General managers have the task of shaping the whole, of manipulating the informal to achieve formal goals, of reshaping the official so that it more adequately reflects empirical realities and potentialities. Although their work involves an enormous number of highly concrete tasks, it also consists of high-level, abstract reflection. Managers are continually analysing and reanalysing the organization in the light of new data. Part of that data comes in the form of numbers, available either from routine statistics or else from specially commissioned quantitative studies. But many other things of equal importance cannot readily be measured. For these matters, the manager must conduct a very different type of research. He or she walks the patch, chats with other staff, goes to meetings, scrutinizes documents, watches how others behave, swaps notes with friends and other observers; in short, uses qualitative methods to get at all those many parts that numbers cannot always reach – the feel of personalities, relationships, emotions, language, politics, customs, the comedy and the pathos, the mundane and the exotic, the real and the formal structures, the actual and the claimed behaviour, the whole and not just the part. In academic jargon, managers, like anthropologists, conduct a form of 'ethnography'.[6]

Of course, different topics require different ethnographic techniques. A ward sister, or the manager of a cottage hospital, can live among their subjects and watch their behaviour from day to day. But the manager of a whole region or a nurse who gives advice to an entire district must do things rather differently. Their fiefdoms are too large, too complex and too remote for them to be available primarily by observation. They watch what they can but the larger their remit grows, the more they are dependent on others – on 'native' informants, on shrewd observers of those matters to which they have little access themselves.

This research faced the same constraints. An organization as big as a district health authority was far too large to be studied by purely observational methods. Those who research such matters are crucially dependent on the descriptions of others. Such dependence renders social science a most peculiar affair. In the natural sciences, observation of the data, and reflection upon it, is a matter solely for the scientist. Electrons cannot give physicists a helping hand; algae never talk back. But all human beings are social scientists – of a kind – and have to be, simply to get by in life. So, in some forms of social inquiry, the objects of the study simultaneously serve as fellow researchers, as unpaid colleagues.

But although such assistance is essential, research methods which use interview data pose great analytic problems. Systematic observation, when conducted by the scientist alone, has some very great strengths. Precise descriptions may be given of actual behaviour. But interview talk is a different matter. How can you be sure that people are telling the truth? How much do they actually know and how selective is their recollection? May not the very mode of research contaminate the data? When we talk about others, we often exaggerate, both to make a good story and to bolster our own position. Besides, our views change. Managers who were caught up in the first enthusiasm for Griffiths might have told a rather different story a year or two later.

What, then, can a study based on such data reveal? Two answers may be given. One aim is to capture a new culture in the making; the moment of enthusiasm, the spirit of that time in the mid-1980s when NHS general management was born. Whatever the ultimate realities may turn out to be, here at least is the initial dream. The second aim is more ambitious. Since managers were obliged to think deeply about the NHS, interviewing them forced the researchers to do the same. This study, then, is also a meditation, not just upon Griffiths but upon the way health care is, could and should be organized.

This makes the book different from conventional sociological ethnography. Ethnographers are mostly at a distance from those whom they research. Academic ethnographies focus mainly on the unusual or the taken for granted. Their authors' gaze rests either on alien ways of life – on a strange tribe or distant subculture – or else on some feature of everyday life that we all simply assume – and thereby ignore – until its inner workings are carefully exposed. In the ethnography of medical organization, for example, some of the classic studies centre on features that, though powerfully present, have never before been systematically explored. Studies such as Roth on 'careers'[7] and Goffman on 'total institutions'[8] focus on aspects of hospital or agency organization that were, in an important sense, discovered by ethnographic research. Such analyses also are written primarily for an academic audience. Though empirically based and containing fundamental lessons about health care, they are still addressed to those whose tasks are wholly, not merely partially, intellectual.

This study is different. As a policy ethnography, it draws not upon one but on several different disciplines. Its principal sources lie in sociology, but it draws in various (no doubt crude) ways on history, economics, administrative science and health services research. Its subjects were different, too. They were approached, not as sources of data, but as experts. When asked to talk, they spoke of matters to which they had devoted a good part of their working lives and about which they continually reflected: in public meetings, in committees or in informal discussions with colleagues. Indeed, at the moment they were interviewed – a time when the whole service was being reorganized – that reflection had reached a pitch of intensity that it may never have previously achieved.

Managers had other qualities unusual in a sociological study. Everyone may be a social scientist of a sort, but their theory and method stem typically from that folk science which, for all its great virtues, is so different from its distant academic cousin. Most managers, however, had been trained, at least partly, in the academic branch. Management theory is a part of social science and managers' talk was shot through with its jargon. Consider the opening words of a speech given by a manager at the same conference from which we quoted extensively at the beginning of this chapter:

For those who are sociologists or anthropologists, this is an ethnography. For those with less honourable backgrounds (*laughter*) an ethnography means telling it like it is.

If managers were unusual subjects for research, we ourselves had a most unusual relationship to them. If the people studied by ethnographers are usually quite detached from social science, most ethnographers, in their turn, are somewhat detached from the lives of their subjects. Again, this was hardly the case here. One of us had spent some time as a health services manager; both of us had studied many aspects of health service organization; both held strong views about it; both of us, finally, could quite well have been doing some of the jobs we were trying to study. Some academics had, indeed, been recruited into the new health service management. Thus, although there were many crucial areas about which we had much to learn, on some matters we were as expert as anyone to whom we spoke.

Our interviews, when they went well, thus took a rather special form; they were not just an interview with question and answer, but a dialogue – a shared attempt to grapple with the extraordinary complexities of health care and its management, a joint effort to understand both the old world of the new NHS and the new vision promised by Griffiths. This book is a product of that dialogue and of its varying agreements and disagreements. Sometimes we present the views of managers, at other times we comment upon them. Sometimes we report a district's eyeview of the world, a view refracted through its own preoccupations and responsibilities. Sometimes we simply stand alongside those at district and say what we saw, looking over their shoulders but not through their eyes. Sometimes we take immediate issue with assertions with which we disagree; at other times we let things pass for the moment, returning to the topic in another chapter or part of the book.

The constantly shifting viewpoint, the policy focus, the fact that both we and the managers were experts give our ethnography an unusual form. One final feature deserves comment: our heavy reliance on extensive quotation. All ethnographies depend upon speech but many use only the occasional, judicious extract to make a point. Here, however, where managers were experts and the NHS was so vast and varied, only detailed quotation could hope to give a real flavour of Griffiths and the organization it sought to transform. But lengthy quotation is a tricky medium to use. Extracts may be individually gripping but prove overwhelming in aggregate. The next chapter, therefore, prepares the reader for what is to come through a close rehearsal of some of the book's main arguments. In it, we set Griffiths in historical context and outline the problems that it sought to overcome and the methods that it hoped to use.

# 2 NHS management: history and background

The NHS, as created in 1948, was brilliant but partially flawed: brilliant because it offered real and politically viable solutions to many of the key problems in paid health care delivery; flawed because, faced with the rampant power of the medical profession, it failed, for nearly forty years, to establish a proper management structure and an integrated corporate culture. Such failures were the main justification for Griffiths, but before Griffiths can be understood some grasp of the traditional NHS is essential. This, in its turn, requires some consideration of the key issues in health care. We therefore start with the dilemmas which face all modern health care systems, then proceed to an analysis of the old NHS, reviewing its structure, history, achievements and failures. The story is somewhat lengthy, but managers' views on the new NHS cannot be understood without careful consideration of what went before.

## The peculiarities of health care organization

Several features, taken together, distinguish health care from any other sphere of human endeavour. Life is the precondition of all human action. Perhaps because of this, health care provision is among the most intricate of all human phenomena. Here is the quintessential interface of the biological and the social realms, both of them extraordinarily complex and in their interaction doubly so. Such complexity has three crucial consequences. The first two effects form a pair. On the one hand, most patients know little of medical practice. On the other, despite all the advances of medical science, doctors themselves are often ignorant and ineffective in their dealings with disease. We are mortal and likely to remain so. Most health care is merely palliative, not curative. Finally, because the bio-social realm is so complex, an enormous variety of health and social services is required, and so also is massive input from both the natural and the social sciences.

All this creates some fundamental dilemmas. The first concerns the weak position of the client of paid health care. Despite the uncertainty of what care can offer, people's need for good health and their ignorance of bio-medicine implies a major potential dependence on those who service their needs. The very nature of the service means that crucial sections of the client population are in no fit state to look after their own interests. The concrete form that health care takes is thus profoundly shaped by those who supply it. In the language of economics, supplier-induced demand is a characteristic feature of all health care systems.

If the first conundrum concerns the control of health care, a second set of dilemmas centre on finance.[1] Because health is so crucial and disease is so complex, our demands upon health care are potentially infinite. That care, in its turn, is enormously expensive and modern health care is particularly so. Because disease incapacitates, health services are labour intensive. Because disease is so complex it can also, at least in a modern society, make extraordinary demands upon technology. Moreover, those who most need care – the dying, the seriously ill and those crippled in body or mind – often cost most to care for and yet are least able to pay.

Finally, the many forms that illness can take, the many sciences that may be called on and the huge variety of modes of life in a modern society, all produce, in their turn, enormously complex health care provision. Every modern health system consists of an unevenly scattered army of different specialisms and trades, all requiring systematic coordination if just the right service is to be provided for each patient.

## The NHS solution

If that is the quandary, what is the solution? The NHS, as originally conceived, cut through a good many of these dilemmas. Where some other health systems groaned under the strain, the NHS offered practical, sensible answers to many of the core problems that face modern health systems. The care that it made available was available to all (more or less). The NHS was a state organization which could be organized to serve all the population. Freed from the contingencies of local history and parochial vision, a national service might be planned to coordinate all its resources in the most fruitful way. At the same time, the care that the NHS provided was paid for through taxation and was thus free at the point of delivery. Such financial arrangements served the patients in more than one way. The concerned, committed and thus eager suppliers of an often uncertain health care were strictly controlled through two key devices: the abolition of 'fee for service' and the availability of consultant care only through GP referral. These points need some brief elaboration, for they are crucial to the argument that is to follow.

Where doctors are paid directly for each item of service, they seem, so the evidence suggests, to intervene far more than is actually necessary. The NHS prevented this, on the one hand by paying a salary to hospital doctors and, on the other hand, by giving an income to GPs which was based on the number of patients who had registered with them, not on the individual services they provided. NHS doctors still, as we shall see, possessed enormous individual power, but the NHS had removed the purely financial incentives to cut and to dose which plague all insurance-based systems. Fee for service systems are, in fact, extraordinarily expensive. Their vastly increased cost is made up of three components: the social cost to the patient of unnecessary treatment; the immediate financial cost to the patient, the company or the taxpayer, of the medical intervention; and the huge cost to the health care system of the elaborate billing and reimbursement administration that is needed where each item of service is individually paid for. The NHS was much cheaper, much simpler and – so most commentators argued – just as effective in the health care it provided.

It had other economic virtues too. In all modern health care systems, hospital doctors control access to the most expensive items, both to the high technology and, above all, to hospital care – nursing is the single largest item of health service expenditure. But in the NHS, unlike most other countries, patients could reach a hospital only if they had first been referred by a general practitioner: GPs had a monopoly on most primary care. Expensive, often uncertain, hospital treatment was therefore based on at least two medical opinions, not just one. This sensible device had its origins in nineteenth-century demarcation disputes between GPs and hospital outpatient departments. In most other countries, the hospitals won. The battle over primary care led to a slow but terminal decline for general practice. In Britain, however, a gentlemen's agreement was reached which allowed each branch of the trade to prosper. Through this historical accident which took place long before its birth, the NHS had yet a further barrier to unnecessary – and costly – intervention.

Finally, consider the virtues of a nationally organized service. All industrialized countries face huge problems with the coordination and distribution of health care. Many conditions call for a welter of different services: some based at home, others in hospital; some provided by doctors, others by nurses, yet others by social workers. Ensuring that patients get a service which suits their particular needs is extraordinarily complex. Not only are there huge problems with liaison between different trades and organizations, but not all these services are available locally. Some require unusual skills or rarely used and expensive technology. Others are dependent on a host of historical, political and social contingencies. There are some areas where doctors like to work, others where they do not; some areas where local charity, wealth or initiative has created a service, many others where it has not.

A nationally organized service, such as the NHS, could not solve all these problems but it possessed the ability, unlike most others, to make serious advances. Take one example, that of distribution. One of the first and most fundamental tasks that faced its creators was to divide the service into different geographical units which could serve as basis for both national and local planning. In England, for example, the hospital service was split into 'regions', while Northern Ireland, Scotland and Wales each constituted a separate, roughly parallel division. Once this had been established, the way was clear for the planning, coordination and improvement of local services.

The task was enormous but over the decades many important advances were made. At the inception of the NHS, modern facilities were very unequally distributed across the country. Some areas were richly resourced, others poorly provided for. The 1960s, however, saw the creation of a major plan for the acute hospitals. Large, district general hospitals (DGHs) were to be built equipped with modern medical specialities, each serving a defined local population. To further improve medical technique, each region came to have its own medical school (before this, teaching hospitals had been concentrated mostly in Scotland and in London and many parts of the country had been remote from the latest advances).

The 1970s saw further improvements. Whereas the original NHS had focused primarily on vertical organization, systematic attention was now paid to the links between each of its many constituent parts. Thus, regions were now divided into 'districts', each based around a DGH but also running other local medical services such as psychiatric hospitals and community nursing. Since the service had traditionally been dominated by the acute sector, systematic efforts were now made to shift resources to the community and to long-term care. To coordinate the vast social services with those run by the NHS, a further geographical division was created between regions and districts which matched local authority boundaries. 'Areas', as they were called, could now start to weld the welfare state together in ways that had never before been possible.

Finally, new formulae were created to allocate money from Whitehall to the regions and from regions to districts. The most famous of these was RAWP, the acronym for the Resource Allocation Working Party which devised the system for assessing regional need in England. It, like its equivalents elsewhere, tried to assess the needs of each tier on the basis of mortality as well as population. Such formulae had a profound effect. Previous funding had been based largely on historical precedent, so the rich stayed rich and the poor stayed poor. Now a huge transfer of resources began. Some regions and districts endured major cuts. Others experienced a major transfusion of resources. Compared to most other countries, the NHS began to achieve a remarkable geographical equality in the distribution of its resources.

The NHS was, therefore, a substantial success. Shifting the emphasis from the acute sector proved hard, liaison with social services was enormously complex but, none the less, national planning, the abolition of fee for service and the maintenance of a distinct body of general practitioners all had tremendous value. The NHS was reasonably fair, reasonably effective (as these things go) and extraordinarily cheap; a combination of qualities that endeared it to most clients and political parties for nearly forty years, despite great changes in demography and disease, technology and the standard of living. Some problems, however, remained.

## Problems with the solution

If the overall strategy was brilliant, there were still serious snags. The same devices which made for success were also the cause of some fundamental dilemmas. For a start, though the NHS was cheap, its frugality depended on the strict rationing of hospital care, upon the barriers created by general practice and on the abolition of fee for service. As such, lengthy waiting lists were inevitable – and a constant source of complaint. Moreover, although care was made available to all, the NHS offered little choice. Again, the system was moderately fair and extraordinarily frugal. Everyone could have a GP, but the dissatisfied customer could find it very hard to change. Likewise patients could not select which consultant they saw if they needed hospital care and though a second opinion was always nominally available, in practice only the boldest or the best connected took advantage of this right. In consequence, so research has shown, the system offered a polite, but fairly impersonal service in which patients were clearly subordinate. By contrast, fee for service systems had many grave difficulties but gave the illusion, if not the reality, of greater client control.

Putting this in Hirschman's terms, client power within the NHS was, therefore, based on 'voice', not on 'exit'.[2] Patients could influence the organization only through public and political means of representation, not by taking their custom to another supplier. Such representation took place mainly at a national level. Various local methods were tried over the years, but all faced many serious problems. Above all, the creation of a national service in 1948 had destroyed the municipal control of health care that had been built up over one hundred years. The local members of health authorities mostly governed only in name. For all its manifold variety, the NHS was centrally run. As a result, so many feared, it was all too often a vast, impersonal bureaucracy.

If centralized political control could lead to problems, so also could the principle of direct financing by central government. This too, whatever its other advantages, had several major drawbacks. Treating more patients increased costs but, under cash limits, had no effect upon revenue. Without fee for service, little was known about the cost of each item of care. Above all, perhaps, capital funding had been subject, not so much to the service's own internal needs, but to the circumstances of national economic management. Thus, many parts of the health service still functioned in peeling, elderly, infirmaries, vast Victorian asylums or ancient poor law hospitals. A national service enabled a national hospital plan, but its execution depended entirely on national politicians and their willingness to spend the money.

Finally, and perhaps above all, there was the enormous power of the medical profession. That power has moulded every health care system in the Western industrialized world, regardless of its methods of organization. The anonymity of the service, the long waiting lists, the problems with capital funding and local representation were all part and parcel of the NHS; the vices that went with its many great virtues. But problems with doctors were universal. However, although medical dominance posed huge problems for each Western nation's attempts at modern health care management, that power took specific national forms. The NHS was based on a distinctive settlement with the British medical profession; a settlement that stemmed from the special characteristics acquired by British medicine over the previous two centuries.

When the post-war Labour government came to negotiate with the doctors at the creation of the NHS, the profession was split into very different groups with strikingly different terms and conditions of employment. General practice was the equivalent of running a small shop. Each practitioner was an independent businessman (most doctors were men) who worked, for the most part, quite separately from the hospital service. Hospital doctors were a far more varied bunch. The most prestigious normally worked in the 'voluntary' hospitals, which were largely eighteenth-century charities in origin. Such hospitals were governed by boards of trustees, but there was no overall boss and the medical staff held enormous, independent power. For their colleagues in the municipal hospitals, however – much the largest part of the hospital sector – matters were very different. These services were ruled by local politicians and, more immediately, by a doctor who was also a manager with very considerable powers: the medical officer of health.

Such facts proved important. The NHS was born in the face of considerable opposition from the main medical trade union. To win over the doctors, deals had to be made, and the price of medical support was high. The Labour government made two fundamental sorts of compromise. GPs became independent contractors to the NHS and continued to practice as small, largely independent businessmen, receiving a capitation fee for each patient on their list. The central management of general practice was largely nominal and remained wholly distinct from the complex structures created for the hospital service. Here too, however, the doctors got a very good deal. Unlike GPs, consultants were paid on a salaried basis, but they were ruled on the voluntary not the municipal model. No hospital had a boss; no doctor had a manager. The privileges of the elite were, thus, extended throughout the whole sector. No hospital doctor need now bend to local politicians or to a medical officer of health. In consequence, although the NHS claimed some formidable powers over the profession as a whole, its ability to control individual doctors was severely limited. Fee for service had been abolished, but discipline was another matter. One American commentator, writing some decades after the NHS had been established, noted the profound differences from the United States:

> The English doctor who is not in a training grade is in many ways more independent than his American counterpart. The consultant receives in effect a life-time appointment and cannot be disciplined except for major transgressions. The GP has independent contractor status, but unlike most contractors his performance is not reviewed.[3]

The effects were dramatic. Though hospital matrons commanded their nurses and district treasurers gave orders to their clerks, in post-war British medicine there were no subordinates at all. Once British doctors had qualified as GPs or consultants they were all nominally equal and fiercely independent. British medical organization was, thus, fundamentally syndicalist in nature.[4]

Syndicalism is a special form of craft or occupational power in which the workers try to regulate their work for themselves. Though its origins went back to the mediaeval guilds, its most successful modern forms lay not in the manual but in the middle-class trades. Lawyers, teachers and doctors all claimed the right to manage their own affairs. In each trade, a lengthy period of subordination and initiation into the mysteries of the craft was followed, once training was over, by a state of very considerable occupational autonomy. Each qualified craftsman and woman was an independent practitioner, who used his or her individual judgement in whatever way was thought best. No outsider, whether client or government, possessed the competence to judge their practice; and no insider needed to do so because practice was, in key measure, a matter of judgement as well as of skill. Medicine, which coupled a high level of technical knowledge with great and persisting uncertainty, fitted the model perfectly.

But syndicalism was not just a matter of individual independence. It was also a matter of a craft, of a band of brothers and sisters, bound together by their long initiation, common practice and shared technical knowledge. Collectively, therefore, medicine was profoundly separate from its colleagues in the service, turned in on itself and its own values, careers and rewards. Moreover, although there was huge internal variation in the prestige of its many different branches, it was, none the less, suffused by a fierce, internal egalitarianism. Surgeons might rank higher than venereologists, but a pox doctor was still a doctor.

Every occupation can have syndicalist dreams, but in most trades and at most times, such aspirations remain simply that. The NHS, however, made dreams come true, at least for the doctors. In return for their support, the right to syndicalist organization was extended throughout the medical profession. That right had two profound consequences for the NHS. At the local level, the service was ruled, not by a single manager, but by the collective power of individual medical preference. At the same time, that collective preference fostered, even enhanced, the major divisions which the NHS had inherited from the past. Nursing remained subordinate and of little interest or concern, despite its huge size. General practice and the hospital sector remained fundamentally separate, each with their own form of organization. Acute hospitals took preference over long-term institutions. Community care remained a backwater. Teaching hospitals long had their own organization, quite separate from the rest of the NHS.

Thus, for all its major successes, the NHS still had many fundamental problems. Access, finance, control, coordination and personal service all presented difficulties. In the mid-1970s and then throughout the 1980s, successive governments tried to solve these through increasingly radical reorganization. The methods they introduced and the structures they devised were taken, in large part, from the world beyond health care, from commercial and industrial management.

## The 1974 reorganization

1974 saw the first of these major reforms. The NHS was given a new corporate structure, devised in key part by management consultants and modelled on modern business lines. A host of innovations were tried. As we have seen, new layers of management – the area and district tiers – were inserted between regions and hospitals and local institutions clustered together. In the process, some old anomalies were sorted out. Teaching hospitals lost their previous independent status and were placed firmly inside the regional and district structure. The last remnants of municipal health care were transferred to the NHS, as community health services became integrated into the new districts along with the whole local hospital sector.

The new management tiers had, in turn, a new management ethos. An elaborate planning system was created, based on current management fashion. The administrative rhythm in each region, area and district soon came to centre round the endless construction and varying cycles of detailed plans. To make these new plans a new sort of staff was needed. Each tier had a management team and, so too, did the key clinical trades. Both medicine and nursing now had a new administrative cadre, planners and leaders taken from within the clinical professions but trained in the new management skills that the new service required.

In a previous reform (in 1966) the old hospital matrons had disappeared and been replaced by a new institutional boss, the DNS or director of nursing services. Now DNSs, in their turn, were made subordinate to a chief at the new district tier, the district nursing officer or DNO (also known as the CNO). And for the doctors, there were now 'community physicians', named after the defined local populations that regional and district plans were now to serve. The old medical officers of health who had run municipal health care had a modern NHS equivalent. Each new district now had its DMO (district medical officer).

In short, 1974 introduced some important elements of modern business technique. It tided up and improved some of the basic administrative structure. It introduced the important notions of management training and of management cadres drawn from within the clinical ranks. It carried forward the major possibilities for coherent local planning that were inherent within a national service. It also improved local representation: community health councils and area health authorities were created and facilitated an input from local voluntary groups and a wider range of local interests.

However, the reorganization was still conducted very much within the traditional NHS framework. Funding was still centrally controlled, the same rationing devices were still used, fee for service was still avoided. Above all, although the notion of local management had been introduced, there was still one fundamental break with conventional business management. Regions and districts now had management teams but no region or district had an overall manager. Yet the creation of a chief executive officer at each layer of the organization is central to all large businesses. Every such organization normally has a single line of command which stretches from its very top to its very bottom. One man (or woman) is in overall control. He or she can give orders to all those who work below. Such commands are filtered through subordinate bosses at each tier of the organization, who in turn command their own subordinates.

Command is, of course, too simple a term to describe the complex realities of organizational life. Managers give orders but they are also, in turn, dependent on their subordinates for information, cooperation and action. All business management is, therefore, a matter of complex monitoring, consultation and politicking. But in the last resort – and sometimes a lot earlier – management is a matter of command. The restructuring of 1974 avoided this. Faced with the enormous power of medical syndicalism, a very different tack was tried. If doctors could not be ordered about, perhaps they might, just, join a team. Indeed, perhaps teamwork was the only suitable philosophy for health care which had so many different trades and which was so crucially shaped by technical uncertainty, clinical judgement and that powerful sense of individual duty towards the sick which suffused all the occupations who worked within it. Were orders ever appropriate in such circumstances?

Consensus management was, therefore, the slogan that characterized the reorganization. The health service was to be managed, but its management was to be conducted not by a boss, but by a group of equals, of fellow professionals, each representing the interests of a different occupation. Every district, for example, was to have its district management team (DMT). The DMT was a sort of collective, chaired but not led by the district administrator. Working together the new team would shape the service, members putting their own occupation's point of view yet continually striving for consensus; moving forward on the basis of the interest they all had in common – the patients.

At the DMT's core lay the new district managers: an administrator, a treasurer, a community physician and a chief nursing officer, each the head of an administrative team (and in the nurses' case, also the head of the clinical service). Added to them were two doctors, chosen by their colleagues to represent clinical rather than managerial medical interests. One was a hospital consultant, the other a general practitioner who was needed to liaise with the GPs, since they were outside the formal district structure.

The pooling of interests, the creation of a common focused view, was enhanced by a further innovation. The central task of NHS management was the coordination of the clinical trades. Medicine might be small but most doctors were fiercely independent. Nursing, on the other hand, was enormous in scale. Yet, if consensus management was to work, every clinician had to play a part. The new management teams were, therefore, matched with elaborate consultative structures. Every doctor and every nurse could vote for the members of elected professional advisory committees or if so minded stand for membership themselves.

1974 was, therefore, not a challenge to, but the apotheosis of health service syndicalism. The core principle of medical self-organization was applied to the entire service. Each craft was to be separate, managing itself but coming together to manage the service as a whole. Accountants would manage accountants, doctors would manage doctors, nurses would manage nurses then, through consultation and committees, the sum of things would be coordinated. Each trade was a self-governing soviet and each management team a supreme soviet. Or, in the words of one commentary on the key reports that led up to 1974:

> [With] . . . the idea of separate functional management – the NHS as a coalition of separately managed professions . . . the Salmon proposals . . . and the Grey Book mark the high water point of what may be called the influence of professional values within the service.[5]

The power of medicine was not the only force behind this extraordinary extension of health service syndicalism. Nursing, the other key clinical trade, played a fundamental role. Long the handmaiden of medicine and totally subordinate to it, nursing was now undergoing a major upheaval. Though wholly different in size, recruitment, education and organization, nursing reformers took doctors as a model. The nurse of the future would be scientifically trained and use independent clinical judgement. A new profession would arise to stand alongside – and equal to – medicine; a new syndicalist craft would be born. 1974, therefore, marked a massive extension of nursing power within the service. The new chief nursing officers (CNOs) in each district now had sole charge of the vast district nursing budgets; the new area health authorities now had nursing as well as medical representatives. At long last, nursing sat at the top table. Nursing, too, was part of the consensus.

There were, then, high hopes. Yet, in many key respects, consensus management proved fundamentally unrealistic. One crucial problem was the obsession with bureaucracy. The comment, perhaps, is unfair. In one sense, the NHS had almost no bureaucracy at all. Freed from the administrative burden of fee for service and unable, for one reason and another, to collect much routine information on the activity of its clinical staff, the NHS was cheap and simple to run. By all international standards, its management costs were astonishingly low. But, in one key area – that of change – the NHS was, indeed, extraordinarily bureaucratic. To build a new hospital or close an old one, to start up a service or reform one which already existed, to integrate the work of one department with another or separate the bits out and start again, year upon year and layer upon layer of consultation was normally needed.

Such tendencies had been inherent from the very beginning of the service, but they were reinforced by the 1974 reorganization.[6] Welfare state syndicalism involved the creation, not just of layer upon layer of management tiers but of an elaborate machinery for liaison with every type of interest: with the professional bodies and with the local clinical trades, with civil servants in Whitehall and with officers in local government, with national pressure groups and with local voluntary organizations. Every interest at every level was built into the formal structure of the organization.

Yet for all this the clinical services remained largely unmanaged. Nursing, for example, was not a profession but an unwieldy conglomeration of diverse and, for the most part, relatively unskilled workers. It was, therefore, in no fit state to suddenly assume huge professional, financial and managerial responsibilities. Nurse training had never been taken seriously in most parts of the health service, while the enormous demands now thrust upon the trade required for their competent execution a vast cadre of skilled nurse managers in every part of the NHS. No such cadre existed, nor was much serious thought given to creating one. A survey of chief nursing officers conducted a decade after the 1974 reorganization found that 23 per cent had neither O-levels nor a school certificate.[7] A profession could not be created overnight, nor could a body of professional managers. Many more years would need to pass before such dreams stood any chance of serious embodiment.

There was also the failure to tackle the relations between the key NHS trades. It proved impossible to rely solely on consensus for the integration of such a huge public service composed of so many disparate elements. Professions might claim a general ethic of service to the client and, in important part, that claim might be true. But they could also readily become a narrow, self-serving monopoly. Indeed, the very features which made them so worthy of admiration also led, when unchecked, to serious organizational distortion. An exclusive focus on one's own occupation and its particular duty to the individual client was a sure guarantee of tribalism. Tribalism – a term used by general managers in the privacy of their own conferences – referred to some characteristic features of the health service trades: to their strikingly different culture, history and organization; to their huge fragmentation; to their fierce internal loyalties; to their general lack of any external vision; and to the consequent difficulty, despite their very real commitment to the patient, in providing an effective, coordinated overall service.

Not only did consensus management embody far too optimistic a view of the breadth of vision that any occupation could achieve through its own efforts, but the system grossly misrepresented the actual balance of power between the different health service trades – and did nothing fundamental to change this. Consensus management was hardly negotiation between equals. Administrators and treasurers were weak because doctors were strong, nurses were ignorant because doctors were educated. Thus, above all, the reorganization failed to examine the internal order of medicine. In the Salmon doctrine, there would be 'managers of each major function', managers who would 'control their subordinates, that is give them orders and co-ordinate their jobs'.[8] However, while a new class of nurse leaders might hope, in the long run, to practice a more scientifically based management, in medicine, there was no possibility, as things stood, of any management at all. Doctors simply refused to be managed. The 1974 reorganization might have created a new class of medical administrators, the community physicians; but they were simply advisors and planners, despised by many of their colleagues and with no control over the medical workforce.

In short, the NHS still took a most peculiar form: a giant state organization which was controlled simultaneously both by Whitehall and by thirty thousand doctors. In 1948 one fundamental element of traditional medical syndicalism – fee for service – had been removed yet the whole profession had been granted powers of which many of its members had previously only dreamed. In 1974 the potential ability to plan and coordinate services had been dramatically strengthened yet nothing had been done to confront individual medical power; indeed, nursing had been offered something of the same syndicalist power as medicine.

The result was a contradiction. At the macro level, there was some real success. Despite the lengthy delays that syndicalism imposed, some real planning was still possible and the system was cheap. By most other countries' standards, the NHS was both reasonably fair and astonishingly frugal. But at the micro level, there were huge problems. The power of medical syndicalism meant that little basic information was gathered on individual medical activity. And what information there was could hardly be used for fear of what doctors might say. The contrast with the United States was instructive. There the macro-system was a mess. American health care was rambling, vast, hugely expensive, sometimes shockingly unfair and unmanaged – at least at the global level. But in some local matters, there were real achievements to record. Given their very different powers over doctors and the systematic information on individual activity that a fee for service system provided, American hospitals had begun to pioneer new methods for medical micro-management; methods which were the envy of the lowly administrators within the NHS.

If British doctors could be tamed, there was, therefore, a real chance for change. But who was willing to venture deep into the lions' den? And who could train them to jump through the hoops that an integrated service necessarily required? The answers were to come from a government that treated doctors in much the same way as printers and miners; that was opposed, not just to the consensus established in the Second World War but to the syndicalism that had dominated British life throughout much of the century.[9]

## The end of consensus – the rise of general management

Something of the new government's wider philosophy may be gathered from a speech made by Clive Priestley in 1984, the same year in which the NHS was to be fundamentally reformed. Priestley was a central figure in Mrs Thatcher's attempts to improve the efficiency of the civil service. His subject was 'the well-managed state' and the talk was given to a conference on bureaucracy organized by the influential Adam Smith Institute:

> The theory of the welfare state [so Priestley argued] . . . has not actually until recently included any emphasis at all on efficiency, effectiveness or value for money. This is a very curious philosophical omission, and the fact that it exists is a comment on the relatively slack intellectual times in which we live, as compared with, say, political philosophy one hundred years ago.[10]

The new government looked, in the phrase of the decade, to Victorian values. It rejected, in principle at least, not merely the work of one, two or three decades but of almost the whole century. None the less, it was also profoundly affected by recent experience. Priestley went on to add,

There were consequently very few positive prizes for determined management or cost control. Public services were free, the unions were very powerful and, for most of the 1970s were dealing with a government that was pro-union and preferred to increase staff numbers than to precipitate discontent. The machinery for efficiency in government was either cumbersome or ineffective, and not much improved after the IMF [International Monetary Fund] intervention of 1976.[11]

In health care, despite the fervour of its philosophy, the Thatcher administration moved slowly to begin with. But the first changes were a harbinger of much that was to come. The year of 1981 saw the creation of annual performance reviews: each layer of management was to monitor the performance of the tier below. The DHSS was to systematically monitor regions, the regions scrutinized areas and, each year, the areas assessed how the districts had done. In its turn 1982 saw the first attempt to streamline the structure and get managers up to the front. Regions, as ever remained, but areas were abolished and a new tier, that of unit, was inserted below districts. Management teams now reached down into each hospital and service.

Such changes involved both a concentration of power at the centre and, simultaneously, a more focused managerial effort at the coalface. The sole rationale for the area tier had been to liaise with local authorities. But, while it made NHS management extremely top heavy, integration between social and medical services had proved hard. So areas were abolished and the mechanism for local representation – the health authority – was shifted from area to district. But, even district itself was vast in conventional management terms and remote from the hospitals and community services that it ran. An organization with an annual budget that could range from £20 to £100 million and which ran many complex yet highly distinct services needed, so it was argued, systematic subdivision.

Every district was thus broken down into units, each with its own unit management team whose membership mirrored that of district itself. The division was conducted in different ways. Some districts grouped services on a geographical basis; others based them on particular institutions – an acute unit for the DGH, a psychiatric unit for the mental hospitals, a community unit for health visitors and district nurses. Here, then, was a real managerial advance. In 1974 the principle of horizontal tiers had been introduced; 1981 had created a system of annual review; now 1982 had refocused the organization much more directly on the clinical frontline. But, despite this, the core problem remained; the NHS now had local managers – close to the clinicians and regularly reviewed by the tiers above – but what could they do to actually manage? A report in the following year put the problem like this: 'If Florence Nightingale were carrying her lamp through the corridors of the NHS today she would almost certainly be searching for the people in charge'.[12] The sentence is taken from the document on which much of this book centres: from the official inquiry by the Department of Health and Social Security into NHS management. The inquiry reported in 1983 and was chaired by Roy Griffiths, a businessman and the head of Sainsbury's, a supermarket grocery chain famed both for its financial success and for the quality of its products. The choice was significant. For a century or more British industry had slipped slowly but inexorably behind the international competition. Other countries had economic miracles; Britain had balance of payments deficits. Only in one commercial sector – that of retailing – could Britain still claim to be up with world leaders, still claim a place in American management texts.

In contrast to the reforms of 1974, Griffiths meant business. The earlier reorganization had claimed to introduce modern management methods but had not willed the means. The new inquiry proposed much more radical reform. In 1984 a further major reorganization was set in train based directly on the inquiry's recommendations.[13] Like its counterparts of 1974 and 1982, the key division between general practice and the hospital sector was left untouched. Griffiths, as it was popularly known, dealt solely with regions, districts and units. These tiers remained. What did change, however, and quite fundamentally, was their management. In each tier, Griffiths installed a single leader, a general manager. The NHS as a whole was given a management board with a chief executive, every region now had a regional general manager, every district a DGM, every unit a UGM. There was, for the very first time, a single line of command from the top to the bottom of the service.

Thus general managers, as their title suggested, managed everyone. Whereas the old district administrators simply chaired the meetings of the management team, each general manager was a real boss, in charge of the treasurers, the cleaners, the nurses, the doctors, the personnel department – the lot. Here, then, was a revolution. The new managers' authority had an extraordinary breadth and depth. Some idea of what that revolution could potentially mean may be gained from the following quotation. In it, Peter Drucker, the main theorist of general management in modern business, writes glowingly of the general manager's formidable task:

> There are five basic operations in the work of the manager. Together they result in the integration of resources into a viable, growing organism. A manager in the first place sets objectives . . . Second, a manager organizes. He or she analyses the activities, decisions and relations needed. He classifies the work. He divides it into manageable activities and further divides it into manageable jobs. He groups these units and jobs into an organization structure. He or she also selects people for the management of these units and for the job to be done. Next a manager motivates and communicates. He or she makes a team out of the people that are responsible for various jobs . . . The manager analyses, appraises and interprets performance. The fourth basic element . . . is measurement. The manager establishes targets and yardsticks . . . He or she sees to it that each person has measurements available which are focused on the performance of the whole organization and which, at the same time, focus on the work of the individual. The manager analyses, appraises and interprets performance . . . Finally, a manager develops people, including himself or herself.[14]

In short, it was general managers, not the clinical trades, who were now to decide on the division of labour, on the training, on the structure and the measures that were needed, on appropriate individual performance. The old coalition of separate but equal professions was dead. In its place stood a radical and entirely opposite doctrine. Where syndicalism gave organizational primacy to the needs of each craft and craft worker, general management was founded on a new type of health service trade, the professional manager; a manager who was dedicated solely to the interests of the entire organization, not just to one of its parts.

Indeed, general management was quite deliberately anti-professional. Specialists were essential, but to general managers their very virtues – if left unchecked – entailed major organizational vices. Specialists possessed a parochial, not a global, perspective. Only generalists, so the new doctrine held, could balance the clinical *and* the financial sides of things, could integrate the doctors *and* the cleaners, the engineers *and* the politicians, the architecture *and* the patients; could see the whole.

Connected with the assault upon specialists was a claim that no form of work was exceptional. All organizations, whatever their business, whether they made cars, sold cheese or treated the sick, faced a common set of organizational problems, shared similar concerns with structure, finance and quality control. The professional manager, it was argued, could manage anything, whatever the nature of the product. It followed that the health service did not have to be ruled, as it had been in the past, by specialists in health care, by doctors and nurses and those trained in the fine arts of health service administration. Good managers should be got from wherever they could be found – from industry, the armed forces or the retail trade. At the same time, the search for the good general manager should extend through every nook and cranny of the service itself. Among a million people there must be many great leaders, if only the talent could be found and applied.

Other management changes soon piled on thick and fast. Performance indicators were developed for region and district; experimental methods were devised for assessing the cost of individual acts of medical care – something that had previously never been possible; a new health service training authority was created. But while all of these were technically separate from the reorganization of 1984, each embodied some aspect of the Griffiths inquiry and were central to the new doctrine of general management; all, therefore, were part of the Griffiths revolution. The chapters that follow describe much of that wider revolution in some detail. However, the core subject of many of those chapters is the 1984 change in NHS structure; the key change that created management rather than mere administration.

## The 1984 reorganization

The new structure, like those that preceded it, was complex. First, if each tier now had a leader, the new jobs were made open to all: to administrators and nurses, to treasurers and doctors, to men and women from the business world; indeed, to anyone who might care to apply. The drive for individual performance, however, was to start at the top. General managers were appointed on rather special terms. The new bosses had just a three-year contract: 36 months in which to make good. On the other hand, they also had new powers. Once appointed, these leaders had the freedom to create their own management structure, one that best suited them, the demands of their tier and the human resources they could muster. Whereas DHSS had once specified the precise composition of each management team this matter was now left up to its boss, subject only to the approval of the tier above.

The new rules and new ethos had two consequences: the clinical trades fell, the others rose. The change in titles told its own story. The post of chief administrator was abolished and many former incumbents went on to become general managers. Treasurers, in their turn, were now called finance directors. Other headquarters' staff, long excluded from power, enjoyed a new prestige. 'Works officers' had been a very humble breed. A 'district estates director', with a seat on the board, could be a very different matter. Personnel staff had been weak and despised; they, too, began to get a share of the directorships.

Such changes had their counterparts among the clinicians. Where once there had been guaranteed seats on the board, doctors and nurses were now pushed aside to make way for the new general management. GPs and consultants disappeared from the team; chief nursing officers became merely chief nursing advisors. The new managers still needed professional advice but they were no longer obliged to have professionals as managers. So, the gains of 1974 – the vast budgets and the headquarters' staff – were now lost to nursing. No trade now managed itself as of right. Indeed, at board level, just one branch of one clinical trade still clung on. Whereas – in England at least – the presence of a nurse on the board was now merely optional, community medicine was saved by the power of its clinical colleagues. Every region and district was obliged to keep a DMO at the top table (though the DMO's real power was often now substantially reduced).

There were other changes too. Within the guidelines that came down from Whitehall, the health authorities attached to each tier were supposed to set policy. The officers, the paid management staff, made the plans and spent the money, but planning and expenditure were all subject to the unpaid members' approval. In the British tradition of government, the unpaid gentleman amateur had long played a vital role; a role which the NHS had both inherited and modified to suit the temper of the times. Thus, by 1974, the era of consensus management, the members included several local councillors and a representative of local trade unions, along with various clinical members and people from the professional classes. But, despite their nominal control of policy, the power of the members was, in fact, strictly limited. Most had little political clout. Selected, not elected, from the great and good in the immediate vicinity of each service, they provided some sort of local input; but the NHS remained fundamentally national in principle.

The 1984 reorganization, however, introduced two very significant modifications. The idea of health authorities was retained, although they too were tied in to the new central line of command. Though ministers had always had the power to veto the appointment of all bar the local councillors, that power had never really been used. Here, too, consensus had reigned. Now, however, ministers intervened. For the first time, the centre played a crucial part in selecting the local representatives. At the same time, and much more crucially, a significant distinction was made between the chairmen of health authorities (as they were called, whatever their gender) and the rest of the members. Chairmen were now paid on a part-time base and their role was significantly extended.

Thus, as the 1984 structures came into being, it was chairmen who were the first to be appointed. They, in turn, had a crucial role to play in the selection of each authority's general manager. Moreover, in elevating the chairmen – and in selecting many businessmen for the post – the government created yet another significant leader; one who would work alongside the general manager and yet further strengthen the senior management tiers.

In short, in every tier of the service, there was a huge increase in the power of professional managers. A line of command now stretched out from Whitehall into every branch of the hospital service. Three further points are worth noting. The first concerns the national variations in the new NHS structure. Northern Ireland, Scotland and Wales each had their own versions (for simplicity's sake, our account has focused solely on that which took place in England). The one crucial difference between the four nations concerned nursing. In England, as we have seen, there was no guaranteed place for a nurse in the senior management tiers. All the other countries, however, insisted that each district appoint a chief nursing advisor.

A second point concerns the assault on the old style of management: that functional management in which each trade ran its own affairs. Now nurses could manage doctors and administrators could manage nurses. But the new regime took such interchangeability one step further. Hybrid posts were created which combined two, sometimes even three, separate functions. At district, for instance, the nurse advisors and medical officers were both candidates to combine such duties with a further new role. A few might become UGMs or directors of personnel or information, but many more were placed in charge of district quality control.

Finally, since each general manager could devise a structure of his or her own – always subject, of course, to review from above – there was huge local variation in the forms that resulted. Consider just two which relate to the clinical trades. Nursing might be generally downgraded, but there was much diversity in what was actually done. Some districts swept nurses off the management board, others retained them and, in a few, the new CNA was the old CNO in all but name, still holding the budget and managing the trade. All districts removed purely clinical doctors from the management team; none the less there were some, particularly those with medical schools, where a huge attempt was made to recruit doctors into general management positions. Here as elsewhere Griffiths was flexible.

## Conclusion

In summary, 1984 saw a huge and perhaps irrevocable change. Where once there had been administration, now there was management from the top to the bottom of the service. The old agreement had been broken. In principle, at least, Whitehall was no longer willing to share power with the clinical trades, no longer content to leave matters to the doctors. Yet, for all this novelty, one of the most striking facts about 1984 was the absence of fuss. Five years later, a new set of government proposals that built directly on Griffiths was to cause widespread professional and political confrontation but 1984 was a very different affair. Nurses, the most immediate losers, certainly protested. The RCN ran a memorable poster campaign. But, nursing apart, little else happened. Doctors moaned but accepted the changes. Opposition politicians rapidly gave their support. Thatcherism might be loudly and publicly condemned in many different areas, but not here. A few raised their voices; even fewer were heard. The principle of health service management was an idea whose time had come. The remainder of this book explores those principles and the problems in their practical implementation. It does so largely in managers' own words. From now on, managers speak too.

# PART 2    MANAGING THE CLINICAL TRADES

# 3    Doctors and nurses

General management means, above all, micro-management: the organization, coordination and close monitoring of the frontline. The first part of this book therefore contains a close examination of the frontline in health care. It looks at the key clinical workers, at doctors and nurses. Our account, however, is selective. The whole rationale of the Griffiths reforms lay in the proposition that there was something fundamentally wrong with the old nature and organization of the clinical trades. So our story focuses only on the aspects of those trades that presented major problems – at least in managers' eyes – for the creation of an efficient and effective service.

This is not, therefore, a rounded picture. Our topic may be doctors and nurses, but our perspective in this and the succeeding chapter is solely the management point of view. Moreover, our portrait – like the book as a whole – is a collage and not a picture of a particular hospital, district or service. We have drawn on many different speakers to create a composite account. That account is based on the comments of a wide variety of managers (using a broad definition) – of general managers and nurse managers, of community physicians, treasurers and chairmen. Such managers had one thing in common: they had survived, sometimes profited from, the Griffiths reorganization. So these views on the clinical trades are the views of those who – for the most part – were committed, or not wholly opposed, to the major changes that had taken place. As such, the picture they painted was often selective, deliberately drawn to illustrate the worst, not the best, of medicine and nursing – the horrors that justified, so they held, the radical Griffiths reforms.

In giving their diagnosis and speaking of their many frustrations, most of these managers drew on twenty years or more of health service experience, on widely varied careers that had taken them through very different positions and highly disparate locations. But, despite the great variation in their backgrounds, there were some very striking similarities in their analysis of the problems posed by clinicians. An ex-administrator, now a tough general manager with decidedly Thatcherite tendencies, could hold remarkably similar views – in certain key respects – to a manager who had pioneered the professional development of nursing. Of course, there was sometimes much less unanimity over the solutions that might be necessary. None the less, many of the complaints about the clinical trades – at least as they were currently organized – were very much the same.

This is a backroom view of the NHS and its management. Those we observed, heard speak or talked to ourselves were often outspoken. Why quote these selective, often satirical, necessarily distorted tales? Like a play, our story has several acts and each tries to balance or complement those that have gone before; each part must be interpreted in the light of the whole. Thus, our aim in these opening chapters is not to be fair to doctors and nurses but to present, in its most vivid form, the new managers' case against the old ways of running the clinical trades, the moments of anger, frustration and despair that led people from many different backgrounds to feel that change was urgently needed. Other points of view come later on.

## Medical individualism, medical power

We begin, then, with the managers' indictment. Take doctors first. The old NHS specialized in macro- not micro-management, in the shaping of broad structures rather than individual action. At the micro level, doctors were left free to run things in the way that they wanted and the power of medical syndicalism meant, so the new managers argued, that a rampant individualism reigned throughout the length and breadth of the service. Consider this reflection by a doctor turned manager on his ex-colleagues:

> UGM: The planning system exists in the NHS simply to legitimize developments which have already taken place . . . I'm a child psychiatrist and one of the things I've learnt is that it's almost impossible to get children to do what you want them to do – they're very like doctors . . . One hospital administrator said to me the other day that he was answerable to 96 doctors who were answerable only to God – and four of them didn't even accept that!

Medical individualism was exemplified in every type of decision made by doctors. Consider, for example, the huge range of variation in medical treatment decisions, variations which, as these extracts indicate, were a key topic in the management conferences which surrounded the introduction of Griffiths:

> *[handwritten margin note: Regional gen. mgr.]*
>
> RGM: There was a study in our region of cataract surgery. The variation in length of in-patient stay for the operation was between three and twelve days, with a mean of four days! Yet for private patients the mean was just two days! When we challenged the twelve-days man, he said it was to ensure high quality of care – yet his private patients were only staying two days.

> *[handwritten margin note: Health services researcher]*
>
> HSR: What about surgical output? If you look at the data from trauma orthopaedics, the discharge rate by whole-time equivalent surgeons varies from 0 to 1,000 annually. Of course the data may be ropy. But the probability is that some surgeons are lazy and some are not . . . We have very diverse ways of working in the NHS! And they can't say they're off attending Royal College meetings. Most of those who attend are the hard working surgeons . . . Another example. The death rate from

*hospital activity analysis*

cholecystectomy [surgical removal of the gall bladder] in 51 districts varies from ½ to 4 per cent. Is this just because HAA is inaccurate? I'm not saying it's all poor performance. On the contrary, we have some super performers – but we also have some very poor performance and this question must be addressed. It's what I call grasping the Normansfield nettle.[1] A lot of people know what the problems are but they refuse to do anything about it. I recently did a report for a health authority and they refused to officially accept the data on surgeons' workload as they said it would be too hard to handle! . . . I'm tired of facing my neighbour over the fence who's been waiting four years for an operation. The medical profession has been very slow on accepting measurement. Some things are superb; for example, the routine inquiries into maternal mortality, but in many other things they have been very slow – peri-operative deaths for example – very slow to come forward.

Medical individualism was equally apparent in the distinctive way in which doctors' participation in management decision making was reported. Decisions by the professional advisory committee might carry little weight with any particular doctor unless he or she was also on the committee:

*chief nurse advisor*

*CNA:* They [doctors] may meet together but there is no entity and the real danger I've found, the real problem, is that you send them a paper, you attend the meeting – I've done this on our policy on resuscitation [that] nurses will initiate emergency resuscitation, including defibrillation – yes, the medical advisory committee agree to all these things in the meeting, all the people who are there do. And then you find that they don't disseminate the information through their organization, so the people who are not there don't know that the committee has agreed that on their behalf. They don't have any true representative authority, they are not delegates in any sense, they are not mandated. And you find that two or so years on, you are still quarrelling with individual practitioners . . . 'I'm not going to allow my nurses to put a defibrillator on my patients.' 'But doctor, you might be fifteen miles away, up in the hills. Would you rather your patient died?' . . . You know it's hard work.

The only way round this problem of representation was to include everyone on the advisory committee, but this too had its difficulties:

*DGM:* They won't allow either me or the deputy DGM in there and there are 50 people on the medical advisory committee! John [chair of MAC] doesn't believe in small, exclusive committees!

This lack of interest in corporate decision making was equally reflected, so managers argued, in many doctors' ignorance of management issues, in their inability to understand the new management proposals and in their unwillingness to play any part in such matters unless they were paid extra, something that rankled with other staff whose salaries were far smaller:

*DGM:* Doctors only operate inside their own environment. A friend of mine, the DGM from X district, said that doctors were very intelligent but very poorly educated!

*DGM (ex-doctor):* You'd be surprised how ignorant doctors are about these things. I bet half the doctors in this district don't know what RAWP is.

*DGM:* Doctors in the acute unit think that Griffiths is the worst thing that ever happened to them because we've appointed a doctor as UGM and they can't understand how one of their own colleagues can be making decisions – particularly when it conflicts with the medical executive machinery.

*Asst UGM/DNS:* We have a [mental handicap] unit meeting once a month. We set aside a Friday afternoon to informally discuss issues that arise . . . We haven't called ourselves a formal administrative group because, if we do that, we have to pay the consultant to do it and – OK, it's a very small amount of money – but we feel very strongly about it. Likewise we've devolved the drugs budget to the hospital manager because if we'd given it to the consultant we'd have to pay him.

*DGM:* [We spent] half an hour [at the medical advisory committee] on whether there should be free sandwiches in theatre.

Moreover, not only was there little sense of institutional responsibility among some doctors, or so it was claimed, but some doctors were engaged in ruthless competition with one another for more power and resources. Thus, the clinical stress on patients too often meant a partiality for the patients of the most powerful clinicians:

*DGM:* In general, the quality of medical advice from the medical executive committee is insular and acute biased.

*DMO:* The surgeons are saying, 'You can't cut beds, you can't do that. It'll mean waiting lists.' And I say to them, 'What do you mean? If you've got a dementing 86-year-old granny, we haven't even got a service, let alone a waiting list.' But they don't understand.

Indeed, this competition for clinical resources proceeded, so it sometimes appeared, almost regardless of any financial or institutional constraints:

*USVPM:* In the States – and I imagine here too – you measure your importance [as a hospital doctor], even your sexual virility, by the number of beds you have.

*U.S. hospital vice-pres. of medicine* [margin note]

*UGM:* The acute hospital can't be contained. It's running away with money at the moment. There's a half million overspend. The new cardiac surgeon has been told not to take on more than four patients a week and he simply refuses to do this. They've told him not to anaesthetize patients unless there is a bed in intensive care, but he insists on doing it anyway.

Such problems were multiplied in medical schools. The technical and imperial thrust of acute medicine increased dramatically in teaching districts. University doctors had very special powers. Indeed, they not only dominated the old administration but they could stand up to the new general management in a manner that was impossible for any other branch of the medical trade:

*CNA:* The UGMs realize now that the issue is getting hold of the doctors . . . the real problem over there [the teaching hospital] is that there are far too many doctors and far too many sub-speciality doctors, some of whom have only got half a dozen beds . . . and they all want to expand. If you take university appointments into account, over in X wing there are almost as many doctors as there are nurses!

*MC:* It was largely the London teaching districts I was working in [before]. Bureaucracy was everything. There were little empires, office politics, hospital

*mgmt consultant* [margin note]

versus hospital, consultant versus consultant. You'd do a plan. Everyone agreed to it but no one had the political backbone to do it. And yet these same weak people were the same ones who'd go bleating in public about cuts! Any idiot can close a ward. The skill lies in putting them to more effective use. But expediency and pragmatism are the name of the game in too many places . . . Most teaching hospital consultants are pretty much the same.

*DNS:* One of the big problems is that I'm not sure the new UGM has any more control over the medical staff than the old unit administrator had – because half the doctors are not employed by the hospital but by the university and yet he's still supposed to manage them.

*CNA:* I had tremendous support from the Dean and from the consultants. [When the DGM had wished to abolish the senior nursing post at district.] The Dean said, 'Don't worry, there's no way we'll let them get rid of you' . . . and I still manage the nursing budget – the teaching hospital unit wanted me to do this. [Almost no other CNAs retained the nursing budget post-Griffiths.]

Thus the individualistic ethic of medicine allowed the most powerful individual clinicians to dominate service priorities. At the same time, although doctors might be in fierce competition with one another for resources, this was a game they played among themselves. Faced with an outside challenge, they closed ranks. For managers, the huge emphasis on the right of individual doctors to take their own decisions too often meant a tacit agreement to the following code of professional ethics: to support one's colleagues whatever they did, simply because they were colleagues; to use Buggins' turn as the main principle for the allocation of new equipment; to ignore anyone who was not a member of the brotherhood:

*DGM:* We had an outbreak of some resistant infection. We had to close several wards. There's nothing new about that. But we got into a debate with the consultants who said they couldn't direct junior doctors to wash their hands – they were going from one patient to another in ITU and not washing their hands. What the doctors wanted to raise instead was food and cleaning. *intensive therapy unit*

*DGM:* A lot of doctors have a loyalty to the organization, but a number do not. I find it rather irritating and distasteful that clinicians are willing to knock this organization – but you don't hear a peep out of them that the private hospital down the road transfers loads of patients to us and wouldn't accept an AIDS case. Privately, among friends, one suspects they moan to each other – but you don't hear a peep out of them in public. Nurses will criticize the hospital they work in, but there's not the same hypocrisy.

*CNA:* I have grumbled at them over some of the things they have done. They are very bad at purchasing equipment . . . they are very loath to say, 'You can't have that', so when it comes to actually allocating resources, they don't feel able to tell any other [medical] discipline [this] . . . I keep telling them we can't afford it and they have really got to do better than this . . . [It's] 'You scratch my back, I'll scratch yours' . . . it is very difficult because of course they immediately say, 'We have clinical autonomy'.

*DMO:* The only reason I'm treated with just a bit of respect in this district by the consultants is because I once was one [he had been an anaesthetist] . . . Doctors as a group are an absolute shower really. They're worse than any other occupation in terms of selfishness.

Given the enormous power of medical syndicalism, many of the old health service administrators had, so it was argued, simply given in. Even in the new era, many consultants expected to be dealt with individually at the very highest level. Particular consultants might try and do deals at any time and with anyone – with managers, with other trades, with the chairmen, with treasurers over breakfast. Moreover, the medical demand to go right to the top, the assumption that all managers, no matter how senior, were there to serve them individually, carried over even into the private sector:

> *DNS:* Consultants try and solve everything by themselves . . . In the past, they just nobbled an administrator and went off on their own to do some *ad hoc* planning. Not all administrators did this but some did, because this way they didn't get any aggravation – no doctors bursting through their doors demanding to know what was going on. Doctors nobbled nurses in exactly the same way. In the acute unit, it was all *ad hoc* planning led by individual consultants just nobbling administrators and nurses . . . there were endless little deals going on all over the place . . . and deals could get passed without being debated at all by the unit planning group! Doctors just manipulated the administrator and things happened without anyone else knowing about it!

> *DCh:* What does a non-executive chairman do? One is constantly taking the temperature – being an open door. I would say that never a week passes without two or three people – usually doctors – coming to talk.

> *DFD:* The DGM has just had this row over how many pacemakers are to be bought – in the past the consultants simply bought as many as they wanted. I had a consultant on the phone at eight o'clock this morning, he rang while I was having breakfast. Fortunately Bernard [DGM] had rung me over the weekend to brief me. The consultant was seeking a statement of our general policy here – but he didn't tell me what had happened or warn me he was seeing Bernard again later on today. He was just trying it on.

> *DGM:* What's the difference between the behaviour of clinicians in the private sector and the NHS?

> *PSGM (from an American-owned private hospital):* It's a Jekyll and Hyde thing, the same person in different guises! They do bring over into the private sector some of the old bad habits – and we have to educate them! The first year of our operation I got calls from doctors phoning me, the managing director! They were trying to go the back door route . . . I had to repeat over and over again, 'There are no special funds in my back pocket' . . . You [NHS managers] have got a tougher job, there's no doubt about it, OK?

## Nursing hierarchy, nursing subordination

If managers' main problem with medicine was its rampant individualism, many of their problems with nursing were quite the reverse. While medical syndicalism was the exemplar of the potential power of a profession, nursing was organized on quite opposite principles. Yet despite this fundamental difference, the principles on which nursing was based still created huge problems for management. Where doctors exhibited an excess of individual initiative, too often nurses had no initiative at all. For all the attempts to create something closer to a profession, many managers still felt that key aspects of nursing were dominated by an outlandish sense of hierarchy. A quasi-military discipline could extend throughout nursing, to every level of the organization:

> *DMO:* Nurses took the wrong turn at the very start of nurse management. They should have taken the professional role. What we need is nurse practitioners equivalent to the hospital consultant who, like doctors, would have peers. They could be managed either by nurses or non-nurses. But, instead, nursing got trapped in the strange blind alley of a hierarchical system where to get any money you had to go up the bureaucracy. But nurses are basically staff, not line.

*nursing & midwifery*
*prof. advisory cttee*

> *INT:* Why didn't you appoint a CNA but rather let one be elected by the NMPAC?
> *DGM:* The previous CNA had had a bad effect on nurse management all the time that I'd been in the district. I felt I had first to get the nurse managers' confidence back. It's taken nurses some time to realize what peer group support is. They've needed time to develop their confidence . . . The main people imposing a hand-maiden role on nursing having been nurses themselves . . . And it's not just oppressing other nurses. There's also been some oppression of the domestics. We've got a little problem there at the moment.

> *CNA:* You haven't asked me anything about relations with the RNO . . . The meetings are dreadful! We're simply told what to do. They're a replica of the old NMPAC here. It's the sort of meeting you always send a deputy to if you can!

> *DNS:* [It's being] . . . afraid of failing. That's what I think is the biggest thing with nursing staff. They are so used to being criticized if they lose a pill or somebody has happened to miscount them – and then they have to report it. And they are so used to being told, 'How could you let that happen, nurse?'

> *DNE:* Most nurses come in with a do-gooding personality. The trouble is they don't ask too many questions. This is the hidden curriculum in nursing – open doors for your seniors and don't sit too close to them!

Moreover, although there was a radical internal reform movement within nursing – led by the Royal College – to create a proper nursing profession, comparatively modest attempts at professional development could still meet considerable opposition, not just from outsiders elsewhere in the service, but from senior figures within its own ranks. Many nurse managers, so it was held, positively enjoyed bossing their subordinates and had little interest in actively soliciting their junior staff's opinion or seriously enhancing their technical skills. To do so was too threatening to their own status:

> *CNA:* They [the district's DNSs] don't accept, in my opinion, the professional role. One of the things we have strengthened is the nursing and midwifery advisory network – or at least we've tried to strengthen that – and it's interesting that some of them [DNSs] are not particularly interested in trying to get feelings from the grassroots staff.

*DNS:* There was fantastic opposition to our sister development programme at middle management level. The nursing officers blocked every move.

*DNS:* Most senior nurses are so concerned to deliver nursing services that they don't think how to develop nursing. Perhaps it's because they're so hierarchical and insecure. It's a particular style of management.

*CNA:* Despite two or three years of really hard work, there are still signs of real backwardness . . . still some nurses who don't understand anything about professional responsibility. That woman in the meeting today who wanted auxiliaries to sign for everything! She's a clinical tutor.

This hierarchical world could extend, so it was argued, deep into some nurses' private lives and personality. In those parts of the country with expensive housing, the closure and sale of nurses' accommodation (one item in the new NHS policy) presented major problems in retaining staff. None the less, some managers were glad to see the old nurses' homes abolished. Nurses who had lived there for years could become institutionalized, as could those who worked too long in the same place:

*DNS:* There are a few nurses there [nurses' home] who've been there over twenty years and don't know any other world. It's dreadful. They go very peculiar.

*DNS:* The problem with mental handicap hospitals is that some of the managers are as institutionalized as the patients. You see that woman over there? She's forty now and she's been here since she was fifteen.

*DNS:* There have been two big recruitment surges into mental hospital nursing: one in the inter-war years during the period of high unemployment; the other during demob at the end of the war. Mental hospital nursing lent itself to the military model. It was an institution for the staff as well as the patients – and the superintendent physician was the commander.

All these factors, so managers held, had a further consequence which distinguished nursing quite dramatically from medicine. The elaborate hierarchy, the lack of any developed sense of professional identity and the initiation into submission from the earliest years meant that nursing was extraordinarily weak in the face of external opposition. Nursing might be huge in number, but there was relatively little occupational solidarity – some for example rejoiced in the demotion of the old nurse managers at district and region:

*CNA:* The divisions among nurses are its weakest point. Nurses shouldn't laugh at the fact that X district has managed without a CNO [as some members of the audience just had].

*RCN representative:* The key point made by Jean [the CNA who was the previous speaker] is that there are groups of speakers who are not supporting their CNO. We're much more cruel to each other as a profession than the other professions in the health service; indeed than most other professions I know of.

As a result, where nurses often found it hard to oppose the new management, DGMs had to proceed much more gingerly with doctors:

*DNS:* All too often in nursing, you start out with the support of your colleagues and when you get to the chairman's door and knock on it and say, 'We're all saying, "No!"' you suddenly find there's no one with you!

*DGM:* The capacity of nurses to screw the system is much less than that of doctors.
*INT:* What is it doctors have got?
*DGM:* Clout. They have the best trade union in the world and a capacity to retreat into professionalism that no one can challenge. There is immense group loyalty. Normansfield was a classic example. When the chief was suspended, they all came out in sympathy, but when he was shown to be culpable, nobody said a word . . . [By contrast] . . . we had a nursing officer suspended for unprofessional conduct – this involved transactional analysis of a very brutal kind and coercion of junior staff. The union went to the paper and said they wouldn't have it, but the campaign rapidly dissipated – the bulk of staff just weren't interested – yet this was where nurses were strongest.

Finally, some nurse managers noted that although nursing possessed its own elaborate hierarchy which stretched, since 1974, through every management tier, its place at the highest levels was very far from secure. However formidable an RNO might appear to a ward sister, her position was far weaker than her colleagues' and rivals':

*RNO:* The doctors here [community physicians] have . . . got all the medical contracts – several thousand of them. We've not got this . . . If you count up all the numbers [of staff at region] there's fifty people in personnel; fifty people on the medical side; a hundred in the treasurer's department; three hundred in administration – and two in nursing. That says it all. [This was after a post-Griffiths reduction of several posts on the nursing side but still gives a reasonably accurate picture.]

*DGM (ex-nurse):* The big advantage that the medical profession have got over nurses is that there's powerful professional advice at the regional level – and there are regional [medical] specialities too. Neither is true in nursing. How far is the problem in nursing the fact that it lacks a powerful input at region, so as a result the districts can't get started?

There was, then, a quite extraordinary contrast in managers' eyes between the individual power of doctors and the collective feebleness of nurses; between medicine's influence at the highest levels and nursing's notional representation; between doctors' fierce syndicalism and nursing's massive internal hierarchy. But having drawn that contrast, it is also crucial to see that the two are very intimately linked. Nursing's hierarchy stemmed not so much from within nursing itself, as from the many powerful forces – medicine, gender and the demands of an extremely labour-intensive industry – which had created, shaped and controlled the nursing trade. The effect of these three closely interlinked forces was to powerfully subordinate the entire occupation. As a consequence, it had reproduced internally the structure of its external domination. Tight control from without meant rigid hierarchy within. Though many deeply resented it, nurses had been – and mostly continued to be – the handmaidens of the medical profession, a servant class:

*DNS:* Doctors want a handmaiden. This is what they want. One consultant moaned to me the other day about the need for change. In the past, he said, his tea and toast were always ready for him when he came to the ward! I thought, 'I wish I'd known that before!'

*DGM:* Some people – the chairman of the medical advisory committee, for example – don't want thinking nurses. He believes that all nurses are good for is powdering the patients' bums!

*DCh:* Lots of doctors regard nurses as fodder for bossing around and nurses – well, I don't know if it's natural or not – but some nurses have a desperate desire to be subservient!

Even the most senior nurses could be patronized – or bullied – by some members of the medical profession. The following speaker recounted her arrival eight years previously at one of Britain's more famous teaching hospitals:

*CNA:* Within a fortnight I was summoned by the medical executive committee to account for my being appointed. So I went before them. I had to wait for twenty minutes and the person who went in before me was the DNS for the acute hospital and she was just berated. They were incredibly rude. She was reduced to a quivering wreck. It was obviously a common practice in the past to call matron to account . . . They felt they had every right to ask me to account for yet another post in nursing administration and just what was I doing . . . I was there three-quarters of an hour and they berated me one after another – things like, 'We don't want American-style academic nurses coming here' . . . though *afterwards* one or two individual consultants came up and wished me good luck. [Original emphasis]

Managers, in their turn, might simply reflect medical attitudes. Doctors were the real bosses and their values could permeate the entire organization, affecting the new management quite as much as the old:

*UGM (ex-nurse):* We had this one-day meeting and Jim [chair] said that only doctors and administrators would be UGMs. He said that all the posts were sewn up and that they wanted a GP for the community – they were interested in X – who was quite keen. I told him that I wanted to be a general manager and he said, 'That's funny, I'd never thought of you as a general manager! We'd not thought of having any nurses as general managers in the authority' . . . Jim said that the only way to lick management into shape was to get professionals into management and by professionals he meant doctors! . . . What he failed to realize was that nurses are managers . . . I have never been so angry in my life!

Most doctors and health care managers were, of course, male, most nurses, female. Such institutional stratification was regularly reinforced, so some female nurse managers reported, in their interaction with other staff:

*Asst UGM/DNS:* My appointment to the local medical committee was for six months in the first instance. When that six months was up I raised the matter as no one else had and offered to leave the room while they discussed it. They said there was no need and the chairman made the typical remark which you learn to ignore that they had to keep me on as I was prettier than the rest.

*CNA:* Before the interview [for DGM] the chairman said to me, 'You don't want to be a general manager do you?' I said, 'Yes, I do'. But I kept my application in –

I wasn't going to be put off by sexist talk . . . The interview was a shambles. The first question was, 'Could I manage as a nurse and a woman?' I said, 'Well, I manage half the labour force already, so I don't think the other half will be a problem!'

CNA: Don't get me wrong. I'm no feminist [but] . . . he [doctor/UGM] is sexist and an autocrat . . . He is utterly condescending towards me as a nurse and as a woman. On one occasion when I asked what my role was at a meeting, he said, 'You're down to do the flowers, dear'.

Such an attitude towards women could, of course, also be held by male nurses – and men held a very high proportion of the most important jobs within nursing. Likewise, given the cultural power of conventional gender roles, such attitudes were not confined solely to men:

Male CNA: It's most important not to react to this [the lower status of the CNA] like a little girl.

Male CNA: What I always wanted to say to them [other CNOs in region] is, 'Come on boys, get stuck in!'

DDR (and nurse): Of course, there is also the gender thing. I am the only woman with a senior appointment at district level. I wrote a letter for the DGM the other day and gave it to [general typing services]. When it was returned to me the secretary had typed in 'Mrs Frances Smith'. I said to her, 'But I told you to put Director of Research at the bottom' and she said, 'Oh! Will you be able to sign it then?'

## Medical science, nursing ignorance

One key contrast that managers drew between medicine and nursing thus lay in doctors' individualism and nurses' subordination (both internal and external). But to fully grasp managers' views of their position within the health service – and their complex relation to one another – one further distinction must be made. While all doctors were educated, most nurses were not. Medicine was backed by several hundred years of scientific investigation and its students had received a university-level education for over one hundred years. By contrast, nurse training was mostly a matter of discipline and routine, but not of science. The radically different education that each trade received was a fundamental factor in their respective organization. Medical syndicalism rested on medical knowledge; nursing hierarchy on nursing ignorance.

Since medical training and medical science are so familiar, there is little point in describing them here. The hidden world of nurse education, however, needs more detailed investigation. None the less, to make the contrast between these sharply separated trades, it is worth stressing just how centrally medical syndicalism rested on doctors' intimate links with science. Doctors were in charge of a remorseless drive for technological advance; an advance which, as things were currently managed, only they understood. All other health service staff, however nominally powerful, depended on them for enlightenment:

DCh: I'm absolutely delighted with the medical staff, absolutely delighted that they're going to have a serious think about where this new technology will take us. Only they can tell us. They're the only ones who know.

For all this particular chairman's delight, such technological progress often generated vast costs, many of them potentially unnecessary; or so many other managers argued. New, highly expensive techniques exploded across the medical world in a largely unexamined fashion, propelled by an extraordinarily potent mixture of individualism, personal ambition, scientific interest and concern for patient welfare:

*USVPM:* As for new technology, we [doctors] don't know how to introduce it and we never have. Everybody's got to have it before it's been scientifically proven.

*Asst UGM/DNS:* A gastroenterology consultant has been putting awful pressure on the nursing staff, so I saw him [about this]. He said that he used to be able to endoscope only a couple of patients in a morning. Now he's got better he can do six! So now he's endoscoping everybody! It's absolutely rocketing. There's a much more accurate method of diagnosis now, of course – but no one's done a study of what percentage are negatives. So now we can have twenty or thirty 'scopes in an afternoon. My endoscopy department used to be part of outpatients. Then we gave up two theatres for this. There was minimal staffing available but the consultant said that was fine – he didn't need any more staff or equipment. But, of course, as soon as he was in, he demanded lots more staff and lots more equipment. This is his philosophy. Get in first and then make your demands!

Thus, doctors' individual power rested crucially on their monopoly of medical knowledge. In turn, the lowly place that nursing held within the NHS rested, for all its enormous size, on nurses' bio-medical ignorance. For a hundred years, most student nurses were primarily viewed as just cheap ward fodder and their education came a long way second to their work;[2] indeed, as many nurse managers argued, it might hardly be taken seriously at all:

*DNE:* When I was a student [twenty years ago] I wondered why all the tutors wore a corset. Then I found out that if you got a back injury they made you a tutor!

Most nursing schools were in fact tied, until relatively recently, to the specific manpower demands of particular hospitals, to the service of local doctors and to the views of the local matron:

*DNE:* Nurse education was traditionally very medically oriented. The consultants controlled the curriculum in the past. They marked the papers, set the exams and chose the students.

*DNE:* In this district there used to be five separate schools of nursing, one for each hospital! When the 74 reorganization came a DNE was appointed to look after all the units and she was responsible to the CNO; so the school became autonomous and independent – before that the results used to go straight to matron.

Despite such changes, students were still used heavily as cheap ward labour. Moreover, the extraordinarily complex funding arrangements for nursing schools still reflected the domination of particular service demands:

*DNE:* Money comes from all sorts of places . . . the EAG for statutory training, the ENB which pays for teachers and non-staff costs, the regional post-basic training budget and the district budget for in-service training and clinical practice develop-ment – which makes life complicated because teachers are paid under different budgets. At one stage you weren't even encouraged to allow a teacher to be paid from more than one budget – pathetic. It's easing up a little now. It was EAG at region that was fussy. District wasn't as bad. But you still have to keep an eye on this. For example, if I have a vacancy in statutory training which it's fundamental to fill, I couldn't transfer someone from a post-basic course. It's daft. In A and E training, it would make sense to employ someone with this skill to teach at all levels – but I can't . . . The statutory training expenses for students who are leaving the base hospital for training in things like obstetrics, psychiatry and community work – this goes to EAG. But if they're being moved for service reasons, nursing has to claim from district. It's a bizarre system. It wasn't designed. It just growed like Topsy!

Thus, though nursing education had begun to achieve some independence from local medical and nursing demands, there were many unsolved problems. One fundamental difficulty was that training depended on tutors who were no longer in clinical practice – and were thus remote from the practical concerns of the service:

*DNE:* Unlike most other professions we have a division of labour between the teachers and the practitioners. This is very unhealthy. Neither can survive and grow without the other. This is the key problem. We need to do both.

*DNE:* [All] this changed over the sixties and seventies. Now nursing is completely detached from the medical profession – which is good and bad. No matter what people say about medical staff, they are realistic. Nurses, particularly teachers, some-times don't talk about reality at all.

*DGM:* I guess nurse tutors are amongst the worst really – in terms of thinking they know a lot (about the NHS) – but actually they are on the side, they are peripheral to what is going on.

*DNS:* The real thing is partnership. The most difficult thing [in this district] was to develop links between the school of nursing and the service side. No one does that. The DNE sabotaged everything . . . If you can't do, then you teach – that's still fundamentally true, which is why it's so difficult to recruit a tutor like Joan, because most tutors don't teach clinical practice. It's not the fault of the tutors. It's the system . . . Despite all the good developments here, we're still working round the school of nursing.

The problems caused by such divisions were compounded, so many nurse managers argued, by the weight of the past, by the sheer novelty of nursing's attempts to develop its own serious educational traditions and by the extra-ordinarily low standards from which many of the new schools had started. The most basic reforms were still desperately necessary in some places:

*DNE:* This school was in a diabolical state when I arrived [two years ago]. It was threatened by the ENB with closure in a year. They had good staff but no cur-riculum. No one knew what to put in the timetable. There was no defined philoso-phy, no aims or objectives. People just did what they had done in the past. They thought there was no time to plan – and although they did have some planning meetings, no action was ever taken . . . My predecessor – who was retired [by the DGM] – just used to put his feet up and watch television. He had a set in his office! He should have been shot.

Even the most active proponents of professional reform might have real doubts about the time it would take to change nursing education. Project 2000, for example, was a radically new proposal, which came from the ENB, the body that set standards in English nursing education. It aimed to take nursing students out of the wards – at least at the start of their training – and make them full-time students in nursing schools that were linked to the rest of higher education. Some observers, however, were sceptical. If, for example, nurses could cling so fiercely to their old-fashioned uniforms, what chance was there of fundamental educational reform?

> ENB representative (speaking to a meeting of CNAs): Well I've seen Project 2000 and I can promise you that by the year 2000 we will have got rid of the hats!

Moreover, even in those schools where major reforms had taken place, many nurse managers still had grave doubts about what was actually being taught. Some argued that in their desire to break with the past, nurse teachers had devised curricula with little relevance to practical nursing care. Cut off from the ward and filled with lofty occupational ideals, nurse educationalists had become trapped, so they felt, in a professionalizing project to ape medicine, forgetting, while they dreamed, what nursing actually involved:

> DNS/Asst UGM: Nurses have lost credibility because they have left the bedside. I argue with Virginia [DNE] for hours about this . . . our nurses are not being trained to give basic nursing care. They're trained to be mini-doctors. I want basic nursing care . . . I want toilet care – that's what I want. We are building nurses now who think that bedpans and cups of tea are not nurses' jobs. I'm sorry to say this. You hear it from doctors all the time that you can't get nurses to give basic care nowadays. What they want to do is intubation. I get very irritated when people talk about non-nursing duties. We've pushed up the entry requirements far too high so that a lot of girls who'd make very good nurses can't gain entry. Girls with two A-levels are a very good thing for the profession – as long as they'll change beds.

The tensions over quality, the division between educators and clinicians and the arguments over the pace and direction of reform were reflected in the mixed views held by some nurse managers of the professional accrediting body, the ENB, and the new methods which it promoted. The introduction to the curriculum of 'nursing models' – abstract sets of principles shaped heavily by social psychology – appealed strongly to the educationalists. They certainly made a change from the more military methods of the past. But many nurse managers still had doubts about the adequacy of the new techniques, as the following discussion reveals:

> CNA1: They [ENB] used to check the dust on the lockers and if there wasn't any

they'd say the training school was OK. But now they check the wiring diagrams [nursing models]!

*CNA2:* The real problem is that the nurse tutors don't understand the models themselves. They simply learn them off by heart and then teach them by rote to the students . . .

*CNA1:* The ENB's advice is crass, they've got no understanding of the service . . .

*CNA2:* In the last two years – and for me in my experience, for the very first time – the ENB advisors have got real credibility. But in general, I agree the ENB has very low credibility . . .

*CNA3:* The problem is that even before the ENB, the GNC was a load of rubbish . . .

## Qualifications and conclusions

Our aim in this chapter has been to capture a few simple stereotypes of the clinical trades, to distil service managers' views of the worst organizational attributes of medicine and nursing – the features that made radical reform so essential in their eyes. In the crude model presented here, the two trades had a strange symmetry, each being a bizarre reverse image of the other. Doctors were men and nurses were women. Doctors were small in number but possessed extraordinary power. Nursing was vast in size but amazingly weak in influence. Doctors were educated and nurses were ignorant. Doctors were wealthy and nurses were poorly paid. Medicine had a vast scientific base, nursing had hardly any. Doctors were independent professionals, possessing a fierce autonomy in their clinical judgement; nursing was not a profession and was notorious for its hierarchy, indeed, for an almost military discipline. Doctors were famed for their solidarity when threatened, nurses renowned for the ease with which they gave way. Doctors were to be skilful, nurses were to be virtuous.

The managers from whom this collage has been drawn were of many different types. Some came from administration, many others came from nursing or medicine. Whatever their origins, there was often remarkable unanimity in the problems they perceived. None the less, our telling of the story has necessarily been selective. We have had to abstract key themes from many different accounts; not every manager would endorse the views presented here. We have also had to simplify. In striving for a few essential features, we have ignored the many local variations that occurred throughout the NHS. Several qualifications should, therefore, now be made.

The first concerns the character of doctors. As we have seen, doctors came in for a good deal of abuse from many managers. Some doctors, so they argued, were selfish, egocentric and greedy; highly aggressive on their own account but always willing to cover up for each other. 'An absolute shower really', as one doctor and manager put it. But, as that doctor also added, this applied to their properties, 'as a group'. At an individual level, many doctors could be fine fellows.

So, for all managers' fierce criticism of doctors, their comments were often balanced by some positive remarks. The CNA who denounced doctors' inability to establish a group policy on defibrillation ended her story by saying, 'But having said all that, they're good chaps really'. Most managers took similar care to qualify their criticisms. As we have also seen, there were some very 'hard working surgeons . . . some super performers' and 'a lot of doctors' who had 'a loyalty to the organization'. The problem for managers lay, for the most part, not in doctors' individual attributes but in their properties as members of a profession. Moreover, even at the group level, their attributes might vary. The management consultant from outside the NHS who had been so angry with doctors in teaching hospitals found his colleagues in a non-teaching district far more reasonable:

*DFD:* On first working for the NHS, I thought I'd find a lot of people who cared enormously but who needed active leadership. This district is like this . . . The consultants here are mostly OK. I've found them positive, constructive.

A second qualification concerns the character of nursing. As the reader may have noticed, many of the fiercest criticisms of nursing came from nurse managers. Griffiths was not the only reaction to the failings of traditional NHS management. Nursing too had produced its own internal reform movement. The 1974 reorganization offered the chance for nursing reformers to found a proper nursing profession modelled on medicine. If some of the nurse managers created at that point simply continued the old hierarchical ways, others used the new powers of the CNO in quite the opposite direction – to foster, not stifle, professional development. The old military discipline was breaking down.[3] Systematic clinical research had begun and in some areas nurses had been encouraged to treat each other – and doctors – as peers. Here, for example, are three quotations from nurse managers who had systematically tried to develop a new and radically reformed model of nursing.

*CNA:* I've just finished three years' research into fractured femurs which shows that there's been a dreadful quality of care – so I had to give a talk to the orthopods and their post-graduate students . . . The research nurses had followed up one hundred patients over time. I showed the doctors that we just weren't getting them to move, we weren't giving them enough fluids . . . They've asked me to give a paper on it at their national conference.

*CNA:* Nurses have become very articulate. We've learnt a lot in the last ten years. We've moved away from being the doctors' handmaidens. There's been the funniest row in antenatal care. It's a real cattle market down there. So we said that whoever actually sees the patient – even if it's the doctor – has to do everything, including the urine! I've had a doctor on the phone to me saying, 'Your nurses said they're not our handmaidens!' I said, 'Quite right too' and put the phone down.

*CNA:* I got permission to set it up [new ward] as an experiment to see if we could get better care cheaper through a mixture of primary nurses, support workers and clerical help for twelve hours a day . . . The philosophy for nursing care [that we want to test in this experiment] is that registered nurses do the nursing. They have individual responsibility for individual patients and everything flows from that. You unbutton the whole of the existing system, including the shift system. You give primary nurses control of the resources and they determine how their patients will be looked after and how their support staff will be used.

In short, just as many doctors were not egocentric and selfish, so many nurses had begun to develop their education and challenge their subordination. Thus, in focusing deliberately on the worst attributes that managers saw – and trying to list these in some systematic fashion – we have painted an essentially timeless portrait of the clinical trades. We have gone for stark contrasts and ignored the internal changes that were slowly occurring within both medicine and nursing. Radical developments in science and technology and the huge growth in the size of acute hospitals were both modifying the traditional models of practice and imposing their own fundamental pressure for a more corporate view of health care organization:

> *DCh:* The sheer diseconomies of scale [of the modern hospital] are very important – and the complexity of modern care. Hospitals used to be far simpler places. Our smaller community hospitals have no problems . . . High-technology medicine has changed the relationship between doctors and nurses.

> *DNS/Asst UGM:* They [doctors] think the return of the matron would bring back organization – but it wouldn't. The NHS has never been organized right; it's a myth. In the days they're quoting, patients with coronary thrombosis stayed six weeks – now it's ten days. So you can't have that old leisurely pace. Certainly in the past the cleaners and the porters did as they were told. The discipline was very rigid. But the same was true with the medical staff. Junior doctors never stepped out of line. But they do now. The whole idea of discipline has changed . . . [Hospitals have too] . . . they were very much smaller . . . You didn't have the big DGH. Only psychiatry had the giant institutions. In years gone by, a general hospital had 200–300 beds . . . Another thing, of course, is the growth of specialities that just weren't present in the forties and fifties – renal transplants, cardiac surgery, oncology units and so on . . . Twenty-five years ago a matron in an acute hospital didn't have to worry about staffing in ITU . . . Specialization puts a huge strain on resources. ITU costs a vast amount of money to staff . . . Nursing now is much more technical than it was. The amount of skill a trained nurse now has to have has more than doubled since I was a student.

But, having said all this, it is important not to take such qualifications too far. Our account has largely set aside the important differences that existed *within* nursing, *within* medicine and *between* different districts. It has focused, instead, on managers' views of the worst of the clinical trades. The accounts we have chosen are, no doubt, both lurid and selective, but there is still good reason to take the main thrust of the charges seriously. Such views were held by many different sorts of manager, both with and without clinical backgrounds. Doctors might be slowly moving towards a more corporate view of things but they remained, so it was argued, individualist at heart. Though its force might vary from one doctor and one institution to another, medical syndicalism still blocked most attempts at corporate planning and allowed the minority to dictate to the majority. Nurses' education might be slowly improving but most nurses remained poorly trained and subordinate. Some nurse managers had initiated professional development, but nursing could still, on occasion, be fiercely hierarchical. The internal attributes and external relationships of each trade might be gradually mutating under the powerful influence of wider social, economic and scientific change, but there was still a very long way to go.

# 4  Managing doctors and nurses

This chapter considers a further charge against medicine and nursing. Like the previous chapter, it deals with the worst, not the best, of the two trades. And, once again, it is also a collage, a distillation of many different criticisms that were made by the new general managers. The further charge was this: although doctors and nurses could look totally different, from another point of view they had an uncanny resemblance – both had so far proved impossible to manage. The new methods of clinical organization created in the previous decade had largely failed. Community medicine had made little serious impression on medical syndicalism. Nurse managers had, all too often, failed both to manage and to develop nursing. Even though clinical nursing and medicine had some strikingly opposite attributes, the consequences for their management were, so it turned out, much the same. The new medical managers created in 1974, the community physicians, had knowledge (at least nominally) but no power over their colleagues. The new nurse managers created in the same period certainly had power but lacked the expertise to use it.

Not only were too many clinical managers either incompetent or ineffective but their allegiance to the wider management team was sometimes in considerable doubt. Consensus management was based on a coalition of tribes; on a fundamentally syndicalist model of occupational organization. The first loyalty of many community physicians and nurse managers had been to their own clinical trade; and those trades remained sectarian in outlook, fiercely attached to their own small spot and with little knowledge of the service as a whole – or so it was argued.

The key concern of this chapter is thus the highly critical way in which the new managers viewed the motivation, calibre and potency of the old clinical management, a management that had been created a decade before but which they were now in the process of replacing. But before we turn directly to their criticisms, it may help to consider just why they felt the way they did. The new managers' accounts were undoubtedly selective, often melodramatic and necessarily shaped by their current position. Despite this, there are some grounds for arguing that their views were far from being wholly inaccurate. That there had been a widespread failure of clinical management seemed generally agreed by almost all the managers to whom we spoke, whatever their original background. Some queried the justice of what was now happening in particular districts, some would have reformed the service in a very different way from that suggested by Griffiths. Virtually no one, however, denied that there were serious problems with the old clinical management. As before, we consider their indictments of medicine and nursing in turn. But, this time, we shall introduce their remarks with some preliminary analysis of the many reasons why the previous reforms had failed so widely.

## The failings of medical management

The new medical management created in 1974 had never really had a chance. Power and prestige still resided with the clinical side of the trade. In a syndicalist occupation it is numbers that matter, and in medicine the big battalions were in clinical practice. Here, then, were the professional leaders, the people who really counted. Real doctors treated patients. Medical management was for weaklings. Community medicine ranked among the lowest of all medical specialities and had found it hard to attract competent recruits or even adequate numbers. Yet this new trade had had real possibilities. Its origins lay in the merger of three different traditions: the old public health doctors who had worked for local authorities; the medical planners who had been employed by the old hospital boards; and the academic discipline of epidemiology. Public health doctors had once run the massive municipal health service. Epidemiology had a formidable scientific base. Health service planners had had a major role in the development of the new national service. On the surface, all seemed to augur well.

But two fundamental problems stood in the way of this new occupation. On the one hand, community physicians had no power. On the other hand, their links to science were far weaker than might at first sight appear. To take their power first, what clout they had had lay in the past, not the present. Before 1948, medical officers of health exercised real power in the municipal hospitals. But the authority and empire of the old public health doctors had been destroyed by the very creation of the NHS. Hospital consultants would not have joined the service if an MOH was to be their boss. The modern public health doctors, the community physicians, therefore lacked any serious control over most of their clinical colleagues. District health authorities might, for example, supposedly plan local services but medical contracts were held at region, not district, level. Local medical managers could only wheedle and plead.

This absence of power was often matched by a remarkable absence of science. Epidemiology was still prestigious. Indeed, its size and reputation were growing. But most academic departments of community medicine were small and some of the leading figures in the academic discipline – the epidemiologists – often showed little interest in management research. Many were seduced by the glamour of the medical clinician and kept their distance from the lowly hacks (as some perceived them) on the management side. Clinical epidemiology, which studied the origins of disease, was exciting, rigorous and often involved close contact with leading physicians and surgeons. Health service research, which examined the workings and effectiveness of the system, was a much grubbier business. Spurned by both their clinical and academic colleagues, community physicians inhabited a half-world. They were not so much managers as, at best, advisors and planners and even here there were many grave doubts as to their actual competence. Indeed, as we shall now see, these doubts were shared by managers as well as academics and fellow clinicians.

### The new managers' views of community medicine

When asked about their colleagues in community medicine, most new managers talked immediately of their failure. If one or two were outstanding, rather more were diabolical. More importantly, while many had a few redeeming features, most had never succeeded in living up to the expectations of the previous decade:

*UGM:* John's a very nice chap. But he's not a DMO. He's just a medical personnel officer, that's all.

*INT:* What about community medicine?
*DFD:* They [DMOs] haven't done it in management terms, have they? They really haven't done it. One or two are different. David Brown in X district, he's very good; a wheeler dealer. He gets in among the consultants. He's very devious!

*RPO:* Community medicine is suffering vast pangs of angst in this region . . . The community physician doesn't know if he's an epidemiologist or a manager and he doesn't do either well. (*pause*) That's not fair. (*pause*) They certainly do the latter very badly at present.

*DGM:* The lack of a real DMO here is our biggest organizational weakness. I'm very worried about relations with the medical staff . . . The DMO is on the medical executive committee only as the lowest form of common courtesy.

*Research nurse:* I was here six months before I realized what community medicine was like. Before I met them I thought people were being unfair, but then I did a stint in the department. All three of them are absolutely ghastly. I thought they were only joking. I thought that at any minute one of those men would say, 'Ha! Ha! We're not really like this!' . . . It was a travesty. I asked about population increases in the district and epidemiological trends and they just didn't know.

*CNA:* The DMO is hopeless. At any important meeting, Jane [DPO] and I have to go with her. She's very bright but she gets off the point almost immediately and gets stuck in trivia all the time . . . Ideally the DMO and the DNO should work together, the DMO looking at medicine, the DNO at nursing . . . but there's no chance of that.

Not only were many community physicians often thought to be incompetent, even within the limited role that the NHS currently offered them, but some were also held to be grossly partial. However lowly their status within their own discipline, they still belonged to the band of brothers. Thus, far from fighting medical syndicalism, many were held either to support it or else to be too feeble to oppose it. Consider three comments from different district general managers:

*DGM:* The quality of the advice from the DMO is spasmodic because the difficulty is a community doctor going against what seems to him to be the power of the consultants.

*DGM:* We had a guy from the BMA down here last week to talk to the consultants about domiciliary visits. We know that some consultants cancel outpatient clinics in order to do domiciliary visits because it's more lucrative. The community physician at region – who's BMA – decided not to record this!

*DGM:* The DMO is absolutely hopeless . . . He refuses to investigate anything. I've been on at him for eighteen months over a problem in Paediatrics and he's just fobbed me off with one excuse after another. He said he couldn't intervene because of clinical judgement. He even said this of the doctors in child health clinics whom he employs!

Given these difficulties – and sometimes disasters – many general managers took a harsh view of this fledgling trade. Formally, the DMO post had been retained, but general managers (and some competent community physicians) increasingly looked outside medicine to help fill the tasks that were once the DMO's alone:

*DFD:* The man here is very, very narrow – just the old public health doctor. He was chairman of the planning group, but he never really did anything. My deputy and the deputy administrator made a far greater contribution.

*INT:* What is the role of the DMO?

*DFD:* What *is* the role of the DMO??!! (*pause*) Another problem area in this district is community medicine. The DMO's been floundering about trying to find a role for herself. She was mad as hell because she thought she should have got planning, not me. She's been booted off most of the planning teams because she never produces any action. She was the chief culprit in the endless delay in the mental illness unit. She produces great strategies, but no action. Her role now is panning out as the analysis of clinical trends. She's a stats' woman. That's important – but why should that get you a place on the board? It could be done by a switched on scale 18. You don't need a medical degree for that.

*DMO:* Community medicine needs a lot more social science in – and you can get two social scientists for the price of one community physician. I tell the trainees we get here, 'You've got to be twice as good!'

We close these reflections on community medicine with some rather different data; data gathered from our own observation, rather than from interview. Failures in medical management had huge ramifications throughout a district. If the community physicians, for one reason or another, could not grasp the medical nettle, what chance had most other managers or health authority members who lacked any training in clinical, epidemiological or health services research? In the absence of powerful community physicians, it might be all too easy for the medical clinicians to bamboozle those who supposedly controlled them. Here, for example, is an extract from a health authority meeting in a district that was faced with a very severe financial crisis and had two acute hospitals, one large, the other relatively small. In the large DGH, the gastro-enterologists were, once again, out to expand. The role of the DMO, however, seemed limited merely to the presentation – not the evaluation – of their case:

*DCh:* Item 9 on the agenda concerns the new post in gastroenterology.

*DMO:* The medical advisory committee want the authority to consider a replace-ment post. It's one year since Dr Brown retired [from the large district general hospital] and the gastroenterology workload has increased a lot over the last few years. Dr Brown's work has been handled by a senior registrar who's unlikely to remain. So the doctors feel that Dr Smith can't do it all single handed.

*Consultant member (from the large DGH):* Dr Brown was a general physician. At present, his work is done by research staff and junior staff. It won't increase the workload. It's work that's already there. In many ways it'll be cost-effective, because we're saving surgery on many of these cases.

*Consultant member (from a small DGH currently under financial threat):* We've just spent three hours discussing reductions; now here's a proposal to increase staff. Apart from the post we already have here [large DGH] we have another gastroenterology post in the south of the district [at the small DGH]. This proposal should be rejected out of hand.

*Nursing member:* We've lost 10 per cent of our nursing staff – 324 nurses in all – but during the same period we've increased the medical posts by 25 per cent and it's all been done one at a time, incrementally. We just can't go on like this.

*Consultant member (large DGH):* It's an important post, we need it and the patients need it. I take the points that have been made but the patients need it.

*DGM:* It's an important point to consider that some new posts can save money. CAT scanning saved 150 exploratory operations. Gastroscoping may do the same. Could Dr Smith [the gastroenterologist in post] quantify this? He knows far more about this than we do . . .

*DMO:* As far as the consultants' posts go, over the last three years, there's been a reduction of five posts. When the senior registrar goes, there'll be a sudden reduc-tion in the number of cases we can handle . . .

*Nursing member:* I would draw the members' attention to the unit management group's remarks that they're unhappy about the need for this post and that the immediate need in the unit is for more nurses in the endoscopy department.

*DMO:* It was the UMG who pressured me into bringing this case to the HA.

*DCh:* But of course – they just hope that we'll find the money from somewhere else . . . This isn't an absolutely straight replacement because we're replacing a generalist by a specialist, so we are justified in examining it . . .

*Nursing member:* What concerns me is that these posts come up one by one; we never get an opportunity to compare them . . .

Vigorous public debate over such a technical issue was rare; indeed, it was not matched in any other authority meeting we attended. Not every district health authority, for example, had such a forceful nursing member or a consultant member from a threatened hospital who was prepared to break ranks with his medical colleagues. In the end, however, despite these exceptions, the result was much the same. The decision was delayed until the next meeting – at which time, after the presentation of Dr Smith's quantification, the post was quietly agreed without further argument. What had happened? In the previous chapter, we cited the optimistic chairman who was 'absolutely delighted' that the medical staff were going 'to have a serious think about where this new technology will take us'. His faith in the objectivity of the medical profession might be criticized by some, but as things stood he was absolutely right about one thing: 'Only they can tell us. They're the only ones who know.' In the absence of powerful community physicians, the medical clinicians all too readily had their own way.

## The failings of nursing management

Even if the new medical management introduced in 1974 was doomed to failure, the outlook for the managers of nursing might have seemed brighter. The new administrative cadres were proud to embody the new status that reorganization had offered nursing. With educational reform under way, the beginnings of a clinical science, a growing sense of professionalism and a seat on the board, there was a chance to show at last what nursing could do. Moreover, one major internal obstacle had been swept away. In the opinion of many nursing reformers, the old hospital matrons were the great bastions of reactionary prejudice within the occupation. It was they, so it was argued, who had kept nurses ignorant, kowtowed to doctors and imposed military discipline. Now change was in the air. A new nursing was to be created, a new profession with a newly professional management.

That management was given the power that community physicians lacked. Community physicians could only advise their clinical colleagues. Nurse managers, by contrast, controlled the nursing budget, nurse training, nursing contracts and the deployment of the nursing labour force. Real micro-management of nursing was a serious possibility. Moreover, it was nurse managers, not clinical nurses, who had the big salaries and most of the professional prestige. Whereas the weight of medical syndicalism condemned community physicians to being mere hangers on to clinical coat-tails, the traditional hierarchy within nursing enabled the new CNO to assume both professional and managerial leadership – this much, at least, was inherited from matron.

However, a decade or so later, although some of the new nurse managers had proved outstanding, most managers outside nursing were deeply sceptical as to what had been achieved, and so too were many of those within it. Nurse managers might have real power but, so the question was asked, how many of them knew how to use it? As with their brothers in community medicine, they were regularly charged with incompetence:

*DGM:* The quality of nurse management was – and continues to be – appalling.

*RCN representative:* The biggest problem we've faced [during the RCN's campaign against Griffiths] has been the appalling nature of nurse managers. For every nurse manager like Shirley Conway that we could produce, they could point to someone who was obviously incompetent and foolish.

*DNE:* It's a laugh the status of nursing and all the hierarchy . . . I feel ashamed sometimes to listen to people on platforms . . . When that person represents you and the future of the profession you think, 'Christ, is there any hope?' If there's to be any future for nursing, the people at the top who don't know anything must go.

As this last speaker suggests, two of the fundamental problems with nurse management seemed to lie in the key nursing attributes identified in the previous chapter – hierarchy and ignorance. The tradition of hierarchy within nursing certainly gave the new managers power. But to many observers such dominance was irrelevant unless backed by rigorous training in scientific, technical and management skills. Proper management demanded both knowledge and power. The problem for nurse managers was thus the reverse of that faced by those who managed medicine. Community physicians had had epidemiological training, but this was organizationally useless without firm sanctions over their medical colleagues. Nurse managers' extensive control had no serious meaning unless they knew how to apply it. Many managers thought they did not. Even the most elementary organizational and financial principles might be lacking:

*DNS:* Regular meetings with the other DNSs are a big improvement. We didn't have them before. It amazed me. I had no regular contact with my boss. I asked for one and was told we couldn't. There was a real block in moving information.

*DCh:* The new DNS at The Royal had his first meeting with the senior nurses and found that he had to introduce them to each other! These are the simple things where good management starts. It's never been part of the nurses' role to manage – obviously it's been part of the ward sisters' role but above that, not really.

*DGM:* Our biggest financial problem over the years has been the continual overspending of the nursing budget.

*DFD:* DNSs are long on emotion, long on service but poor on choice. Do they put the money into this service or that one? They don't know where to start . . . There is a danger that you end up drivelling endlessly on about the profession – Jean [CNA] goes on and on about this – and I don't think I've ever seen her say anything about nurse managers' financial role.

*INT:* What was nurse management like before Griffiths?

*DFD:* Aaah!! Does that answer your question? . . . I've mellowed a great deal but over my time I've battled with one or two CNOs! They always wanted help because they'd overspent – but they didn't do too much to sort it out. That goes for a lot of management in the NHS. Actually getting to grips with things is not much done.

*INT:* What was the nurse management like when you arrived here in 81?

*DGM:* Bloody awful actually! The man who was the CNO took early retirement.

*INT:* Did he fall or was he pushed?

*DGM:* He ran! . . . all kinds of things came to light afterwards . . . After six months his successor was panicking because all sorts of things had been funded out of non-recurring money.

Finally, consider one other such comment from a speech at a management conference. The conference was held during an extensive advertising campaign against Griffiths by the Royal College of Nursing. The most famous poster from the RCN's campaign claimed that general managers did not know their coccyx from their humerus. One general manager had his own, swift reply:

> *UGM:* My outpatient manager's not a nurse. I couldn't find one who knew her debit from her credit!

The new managers, then, were highly critical of the old ways of managing nursing. But although their criticism was fierce, most did not blame nurse managers themselves. Their failures were ascribed, in great measure, to the backward state of nursing at the time of the 1974 reorganization and the absence, then and subsequently, of serious management training and research to remedy this. Far too many of the problems, however fundamental their consequences, were simply ignored; or so they argued. Those who planned the 1974 reorganization had not thought through its educational and research implications. As a result, many of the newly created nurse managers failed to realize just how grossly inadequate their own training had been. In one way and another they had been wholly inadequately prepared for the huge responsibilities thrust upon them:

> *DGM (ex-nurse):* The district we're sitting in spends £25 million a year on nursing. It needs serious research into how they spend it.

> *CNA:* The nursing budget in this district is £15 million a year, yet we spend just £15,000 on research.

> *CNA:* How the hell can nurses be innovative thinkers, given the way they're trained?   .

> *DNS:* Honestly, I think that if we'd had some managers with good training behind them, this [Griffiths] wouldn't be happening now – but we let ourselves down. We have only got ourselves to blame . . . I haven't felt too upset about it [Griffiths] because I feel, well, perhaps we'll get some good management training now.

> *RPD:* Nurses have the greatest potential for general management of any of the professional staff; they've got the networks, the relationships, that are vital to management. They've got the most potential of all the professions.
> *INT:* Why haven't they made it then?
> *RPD:* A lot of them [nurse managers] aren't very bright are they? They're not recruited from university and therefore they've not carved out a role for themselves.

> *DGM:* Lots of nurses aren't very good above ward sister level. There are some very good nursing officers in this district but there are some others that I wouldn't rate highly. It's partly the way they were selected. Salmon [the report on nurse management that shaped the 1970s reforms] was very badly implemented. It was put in much too quickly. Typical NHS. And not enough effort was put into training and selection. The job of a manager is very different from that of an operational nurse. A lot of nurse managers thought it was important to ape administrators rather than develop specific nurse management skills. But the issue is not cultivating members of the health authority, it's developing standards of care. A lot funked this issue.

> *DFD:* In nurse management we have a huge resource – a far, far bigger resource than we ever had with administrators. We tend to forget this. I think of it first as

very, very big — and the kind of training that nurse managers have had is not consistent with that. Traditionally, administrators have been regarded as *the* managers, but in fact, looking at the figures, they were far, far, smaller in management terms . . . [Nurses are] very much the largest resource we're talking about — and nobody puts enough effort into this. [Original emphasis]

To give nurses massive management responsibility without ensuring either sufficient scientific research or adequate management training had, it was argued, had disastrous consequences. Power without knowledge is a degenerate form of authority. Hierarchy became an end in itself. Since it was so important, divisions were elaborated when they should have been reduced. Tiers were created for their own sake, not from organizational need:

*CNA:* It [1974] was a period of growth and no one was made redundant and . . . there was the creation of area, regional and district tiers — a really huge expansion of bureaucracy — vast numbers of [nursing] jobs were created.

*DNS:* We let ourselves down. We have only got ourselves to blame . . . We were top heavy and went from the sublime to the ridiculous . . . We have waffled through since Mayston and Salmon . . . Griffiths has really given us a jerk. I've never seen so many nurses feel so threatened.

*DNS:* When I read Griffiths originally I liked it. I thought, 'This is right!' When you think of the set up we had in X — all those nurse managers — it was ridiculous and a waste of money.

With a huge expansion of bureaucracy and a weak knowledge base, many nurses were promoted into senior management on grounds which had little to do with the expertise required for that particular job. Many nurses, it was argued, became managers simply because they were good at clinical work, because they were ambitious men (so some women said), because they were caring sort of people, or merely because there were jobs to be filled:

*DNE:* Some of the people at the top of nursing really are appalling. They got there just by experience.

*CNA:* As a result [of the massive expansion of nurse management in 1974] poor old matrons' assistants who had been used to inspecting lavatories suddenly found themselves in charge of surgical units!

*DNS:* You get all these fellows who are climbing up the ladder and with no experience behind them. I think that has brought us down.

*CNA:* Some nurses were promoted to management simply because they were good nurses: 'Manage a unit? She couldn't run a bath!'

*DNE:* Other people think we are just a bunch of emotionally disturbed neurotics who get upset about patient care. We've not developed at all since Salmon. We've not developed our nurse management skills at all.

*DGM:* They'd hardly make fighter-pilots would they?

*RPD:* Nurse managers have been tied by their apron strings back to the patient . . . [They] have had a professional training oriented to an individual care mode which it's very difficult to move away from. They don't see organizations as a totality . . .

And this narrow perspective somehow demeans them. They've got a very blinkered approach to their role. The nurses that escape this are damn good. But not many do escape.

*DMO:* I think it's fair to say that the previous nurse management left something to be desired! The DNE was so drunk he could hardly stand up. If he hadn't had an inspection, he might have gone on for years. Shirley [CNO] was an extremely nice, kind woman – God it's a terrible thing to say about somebody isn't it? And one of the DNSs was quite incapable of managing his empire. He had absolute bastards of consultants and the very worst was the one who gave him the most apparent support . . . He was a nice man, but he wasn't up to it. He had no idea of where he wanted to be . . . The old community DNS was charming and delightful. She couldn't manage her way out of a paper bag! What we're discussing here, for example, are health visitors who'd done three days' work in the last year and were applying for compassionate leave! Our new UGM discovered that they didn't know who was employed in the small community hospital. What had been happening for years was that they put all the mad and bad nurses down there and hadn't kept any records! . . . There's never been any nurse management in this district . . . They [nurse managers] had lots of support, but it wasn't the right support. 'It'll be alright on the night', sort of thing . . . No wonder we got rid of the old CNO . . . I felt Jim [DA] should possibly have intervened more but with a consensus team it was almost impossible to solve all this. That's the beauty of Griffiths. The buck has to stop somewhere.

One other fundamental problem with nurse management remains to be considered; one which it shared, at least in part, with its sibling in community medicine. There was, so many new managers claimed, a sisterhood no less than a brotherhood. Just as the syndicalism of medical practitioners reached out and embraced the lowly community physician, so nurses of all ranks, from sisters to CNOs, displayed a fundamental separatism, a desire to keep nursing enclosed and apart from the rest of the service. The new managers' explanations of why this was so depended on their mood, circumstance and disposition. Sometimes this separatism was seen as mere defensiveness, a natural reaction to nursing's weak position. It was also the result, it was felt, of the formidable internal hierarchy which had given nurses little experience of trying to work within a team:

*DGM:* One of the things that struck me over the years was that nurses in senior management positions were spending far too much time defending nursing rather than managing it. They were defensive in a very blinkered way . . . The problem in this district was the lack of any real leadership. What this meant was a lack of involvement in overall management combined with an almost Luddite protection of resources in nursing – a siege mentality . . . People have headed up the profession by being 'a good professional' and not because of their management capacity, which is catastrophic on the nursing side.

*UGM:* When I was in the north-west, I circulated memos beyond the management team – with the exception of the nurses. The reason I excepted the nurses [was that] I did it just once [circulated memos to nurses] and the chief nurse absolutely went for me. I never did it again. Nurses are so hierarchical.

*DMO:* The other thing I do find – and it gets more acute as you go down the line – is that nurse managers want to run their services in total isolation. The classic case here is the community. On even the very smallest issue I have to go through Sheila [DNS] if I want to speak to a nurse on the shopfloor – because she can't bear to relinquish any control. For example, we've got a couple of good girls working on rickets and I wanted to see what they were doing, just where their efforts were going. I went to see them and the reaction I got was, 'Please let me know when you are going to see my nurses'. I didn't respond. After all, I am the advisor on infectious diseases. I just wanted a few facts. If there were any problems, I'd tell her . . . She's just so insecure.

Defensiveness and internal hierarchy were not, however, seen as the only causes of nursing separatism. The new managers argued that the blinkered views of many senior nurses were a direct product of their clinical training; something that they shared with the medical profession. One general manager compared the two trades:

*INT:* Do you get effective advice from doctors and nurses?
*DGM:*I don't think that from either side do we get enormously helpful advice on managing the district as a whole. For example, does it help to choose between spending money on the cardiac service and the cytology service? The answer must be no! And the nurses tend not to answer the questions that you put to them. Where they do tend to answer is on the question of numbers and pay – and here they do answer instantly and constantly! It is difficult to take a broader view if you're a professional. (*pause*) I can't think of any difficulties the district has been in over the last year that have benefited from the professional advice that has been given. Indeed, it is almost invariably special pleading. The wider debate just doesn't take place . . . Alice [CNA] says that nurses are being picked on, but they're not. Doctors are just as bad. Neither takes a wider view.

Nurses shared something else with the medical profession besides a clinical perspective. The narrowness of vision that clinical work enforced was matched, so many of the new managers argued, by a common interest in syndicalist occupational control. Only doctors might have made it to full professional power, but many senior nurses were eager to emulate the style, responsibilities, powers and privileges of medicine. Too often, the assertion of professional status concealed all kinds of dubious goings on and hindered, rather than enhanced, the service that patients received:

*CNA:* We are very low [on staff in the mental handicap hospital] . . . a 24–bedded ward might have three or four nurses on during the day. It's not enough; not to do the things that modern care of the mentally handicapped requires – which is more than just personal hygiene. There's the education and teaching them to be members of society and so on . . . The dilemma is that the senior nurse is trying to maintain 50 per cent qualified and 50 per cent unqualified and I think she's quite wrong to do this. I think you've got to look at different dependency levels and have something like 50/50 for high dependency but something like 30/70 for low dependency, or even a 25/75. And she needs to get that sorted out – she could get another 100 nursing auxiliaries tomorrow.

*Asst UGM/DNS:* The CNA came round one of the wards because there'd been a lot of complaints from patients and pressure sores were going up – we've got a very low level of staffing. She said that in the future maybe we'd need fewer staff – but that they would be much better trained and more adaptable, 'Wouldn't that be best?' I said, 'Fine, but four nurses can't do the work of six'. It's the nature of the work. We need lots of pairs of hands when we're dealing with very dependent patients.

Doctors, therefore, were not the only ambitious tribe within the service. The medical example, so it was held, had spawned imitation and rivalry throughout the length and breadth of the organization. In consequence, both sets of clinical managers – nurse managers as much as community physicians – were often suspected of deep and atavistic tribal feelings:

*DCh:* And, of course, there's now the increasing 'professionalization of nursing services'! 'Oh, we're a profession now and must be taken seriously.' They're all at it – the nurses, the physiotherapists, everyone.

*DFD:* The weakness of the health authority is the excessive professionalism. I found it a real shock when I came in. [In business] I was used to a corporate culture. You'll get professional rivalry at any level in any organization. But I didn't realize how bad it was in the NHS.

## Qualifications and conclusions

We finish with a little shading to our portrait and some general conclusions. If the quality of many clinical managers was thought to be poor, some important exceptions were still made. One general manager cited earlier spoke of 'some very good nursing officers' as well as of some very bad ones. Another, although not generally impressed, considered the few nurses 'who escape' the conventional 'blinkered approach' as being 'damn good'. Likewise, the finance director who felt that community medicine had largely failed in management terms still singled out one man from another district, 'he's very good; a wheeler dealer. He gets in among the consultants. He's very devious!' Another, although critical of community physicians elsewhere, was full of praise for the medical managers who worked in his authority and modest about his own relative abilities:

*DFD:* Generally, the community physicians [in this district] are pretty good. Intellectually, they're light years ahead of me – though at least I've always got my feet on the ground! But if you take Jim, for example – when I talk to him, I feel like a hick accountant!

Thus, although there was general agreement that the new clinical management introduced in 1974 had failed, it was also argued that some individuals had done an outstanding job, had shown what might be done if doctors and nurses could be properly trained and given serious management powers. Likewise, if clinical management had achieved very little in some districts, there were a few where, so it was felt, major advances had been made. Where failure had occurred, it was usually argued that this was hardly the old clinical managers' fault.

Both, in their different ways, had been blighted by medical syndicalism and the political failure to tackle this at source. The might of clinical medicine had long rendered nurses ignorant and made medical management impotent. If serious clinical management was wanted, something far more radical was needed.

Radical reforms, however, could take many different shapes. Some nurse managers and community physicians were highly critical of the current state of clinical management, but merely wanted their own training improved and their own occupations strengthened. Most other managers (many clinical managers among them) disagreed. There was simply no possibility, so they felt, that the clinical trades could be changed without a major increase in central management powers. Griffiths was the only solution.

# PART 3  NEW MODEL MANAGEMENT

# 5     A new leader, a new team

Doctors would not be led. Nurses did not know how to lead. Many new managers argued that not only had internal management failed within each trade, but that neither group seemed keen to recognize external authority. Too many nurse managers were defensive, sectarian, isolationist, Luddite. Too many doctors dropped in on the chairman, rang the treasurer at breakfast, burst in through the administrator's door and answered only to God. What could be done? The report of the 1983 NHS management inquiry emphasized the necessity for leadership. For Griffiths and his colleagues, consensus management had to go. A loose tribal confederacy was no way to run a modern health service. Without just one central power, any group could run riot. If there was no firm leadership, nobody could be called to account. The core of the 1984 reorganization was, thus, the assertion of central managerial control, using the full panoply of modern business methods, over all those who worked within the health service.

The key target of such reforms was that small but extraordinarily powerful trade – doctors. But, though doctors were at the heart of the programme, the Griffiths reorganization stretched well beyond any single occupation. It offered a new type of structure, a new method for creating consensus, a fresh concern for cost, data, merit, quality and patient satisfaction. This chapter focuses on the new models of leadership, teamwork, devolution and performance review, while Chapter 6 considers the hardest task of all – the drive to improve both the efficiency and the quality of the service on offer.

Once again our aim is selective: to capture the vision that inspired most of the new managers who were appointed in the wake of the Griffiths reforms. Having so far portrayed the blackest version of the previous administration, we now set against this a shining image of the new. The black and white go together. Some critics of the old ways of running the service still had serious doubts about the methods that were now being tried. But most managers whom we observed, interviewed or heard lecture were deeply committed to the new way of doing things. As such, they simultaneously spotlit the future for which they longed and threw deep shadows on the past. As we shall also see, most were realistic about the task that lay ahead. The dream was splendid, but its full implementation would be hard. The technical problems with the model, the inadequacies of its current form within the NHS and the many concrete difficulties that districts encountered are the stuff of later parts of the book. Our focus in these two chapters is on the vision.

## A Solomon come to judgement

Most managers agreed fundamentally with Griffiths's diagnosis and recommended therapy. Consensus management had failed; firm, central authority was essential:

> *RNO/RDP:* Griffiths is the best thing since sliced bread! It [NHS management] was a lot of bloody nonsense before! Nobody put their head over the parapet. It was just a talkshop, a devilish waste of money. Nobody took on the clinicians.

> *DGM (ex-nurse manager):* What made me want to get into general management was a porter I passed every day at the main hospital entrance. He always had a fag hanging out of his mouth, he was rude to everyone – he just grunted – and yet, as DNO, I could do nothing about it. I tried but I failed. As general manager I can.

> *DGM (ex-administrator):* A lot of health authorities spent [most] of their time talking about administrative and financial issues – and we were one of those. Now that wasn't through the DMT [district management team] not trying. It was the reluctance of individuals, occasionally, if you like, to sell their wares. I mean, I can always keep an agenda full of administrative and financial matters because there are so many of them . . . One of the most significant changes in this authority . . . is the number of items that [now] appear on health authority agendas that relate to nursing specifically or to medicine specifically . . . I think that's a result of general management . . . [Before] [as district administrator] I could ask the questions, but I couldn't demand the answers. Now, in fact, I ask the questions and demand the answers and dictate – if need be – what the timetables are. So it's not the 'I'll do that when I feel like it' sort of approach.

Not surprisingly, the ability both to ask questions and to get at least some of them answered, to get some action where there was none before, could be a profound source of satisfaction:

> *UGM/deputy DGM:* I go home now tired but satisfied. I used to go home from the DHA languid. But now I can say to people, 'Go and get it done'.

> *UGM:* The extent of a UGM's authority is quite considerable because you take the decisions; decisions that were prevaricated on before. The UGM has authority, the unit administrator was merely the coordinator of a team. It's a very important shift. I've certainly found it much easier with these closure proposals to say 'that's going to happen' – and I had the interesting experience of a whole group of GPs falling in line behind me! That's never happened before!

At the same time, in the ideal model, general managers were not simply bosses. They portrayed themselves as people who weighed the conflicting but parochial demands from all the different sectors of the service, surveyed the district's actual means and then acted. One DGM described his role as 'all about balancing resources', another as 'a kind of arbiter'. This image of a health service Solomon comes across strongly in the qualities of leadership preferred both by the new general managers themselves and by many of their immediate subordinates. Tough but tender, decisive but willing to hear the other side of the case, global in vision but sensitive to individual demand and possible sources of conflict – these were the characteristics that were wanted:

*DDQ:* It's a very stimulating environment here. It's just an enlightened . . .
*INT:* Dictatorship?
*DDQ:* No, it isn't a dictatorship. Jim [DGM] is not a dictator . . . Jim is a *leader*. He's very unusual – tough but open to criticism. [Original emphasis]

*CNA:* John [DGM] wasn't for this post originally. It was his deputy that persuaded him. That's John all over. His strength is his ability to listen.

*CNA:* Alex's [DGM] strengths are that he listens and he takes actions on what you tell him – he's not an autocrat.

*Deputy DGM:* He [previous chairman] had a knack of making everyone feel that he loved them and cared. He would just send you a note, or you could ring him any time. You could always argue with Fred. If you had a good argument – and only if you had a good argument – you could win.

Good leadership meant better communication, which was also just what the NHS needed:

*DGM:* Many of the problems of the NHS are due to a lack of communication. If you compare the NHS to Peugeot in Coventry, there are wonderful communications there, right down the line. They're a shining example. We simply don't have this in the NHS. If they can do it so can we. We have to learn from commercial companies like this    particularly since the NHS is as big as the Red Army!

*DFD:* There's a great deal of emphasis on talking things through and bringing people along with us. Generally a lot of talking has gone on. Dave [DGM] in fact spent a year of his time talking to the nurses, doctors, paramedics, and to my staff as well – to really bring along the new changes. Even if he didn't know precisely what the changes were going to be at the time.

*DGM:* When we came to Griffiths, I sat down with the DNO, the DNSs and the support staff and said 'What do we do?' I gave them the King's Fund document on professional nursing and we got into the issues of nursing accountability to UGMs, what's the role of the DNO and professional accountability . . . We also had a session with someone from the King's Fund to talk through things. [The King's Fund is a charity that specializes in health service management training and advice.]

Good communication, then, meant encouraging dialogue. Several DGMs prided themselves on liking a good argument:

*INT:* What's your relationship with the chair of the medical executive committee?
*DGM:* Exceptionally good – and when I say exceptionally good, I mean we go at it hammer and tongs. If I think he's trying to pull a fast one, I tell him.

Similarly, although one chief nurse advisor had strongly attacked current nurse staffing levels at a health authority meeting – having given the DGM only ten minutes' warning – the DGM commented afterwards:

> *DGM:* Well, that meeting was different to some I can think of! For the first time a chair of the nursing and midwifery professional advisory committee has actually initiated a debate on a major issue. She's finding her feet. There's a major issue there . . . Of course, once she'd said it, there were several members wanting to raise the issue of cuts. I saw the press representatives writing away furiously and I thought, 'Shit!' . . . Actually, I was very pleased that Jane initiated something. For why? It's very easy to get into a rut . . . It would be very easy for me to ensure that the health authority is – well some people think it is – just my machine. Jane has added a new dimension. She demonstrated today that she's a far more effective advisor than the chair of the dental advisory committee or the chair of the medical advisory committee. I like the chair of the dental committee a lot. But if he and I had an argument, I'd have to be very badly briefed to lose. But Jane was super.

So, ideally, Griffiths meant leadership, not dictatorship. Consensus management in its pure form – as a federation of separately managed occupations – had disappeared, but there was still a very strong emphasis on building a team. The difference now was that the team had a leader; for another key argument of Griffiths-style management was that only with a leader could real teamwork take place. Without a boss, the health service had simply fragmented into a thousand specialist trades. Everyone needed to listen to everyone else. Nurses needed to listen to doctors and doctors to nurses; managers needed to listen to clinicians – and vice versa:

> *DGM:* The thing that I'm trying to push into these people is that you don't go out there solo. If you're a manager, or if you're a professional, what you do is you seek advice from the other. You don't go out there solo.

> *Community UGM (ex-nurse):* One of the conflicts in this unit is that Jean [DNS] has real skills in professional development – there's a lot going on there – but her management skills need developing. At some point, the brakes are going to have to be put on professional development – there's going to be conflict. The ADNSs have come to me saying they were overworked; that I was giving them work in conflict with their own priorities and would I back off! Jean's style is very negotiative – mine's not! They've got a free, open process. I want to tighten up. I want a corporate, multi-disciplinary style where the different occupations look at the service together. If I said I'd got £10,000 to spend they'd all want it spent in different ways. I want to see a service-oriented management style.

> *DFD:* Griffiths got it right. He talked of keeping the best of consensus management. That's right. I'd take the view that it is more sensible to have someone take the ultimate decisions – but they'd be wise to explore the implications of their decisions with others – and to reassure them. But at the end of the day, the buck has to stop there.

Thus, Griffiths was, in its own way, still consensus oriented. There had, however, been a huge change. The old consensus had been shaped by a team of nominal equals. Now just one person was in charge. Consensus, of a kind, still had to be reached, but general managers were in charge of that consensus. All kinds of consultation might take place, but, in the end, it was they who decided how the team was to be integrated. The new sort of harmony depended on both communication and command.

## Setting the boundaries

As such, although there was still a team and although the aim was harmony, there were limits. For a start, although general managers might wish to see innovative action and even praise those who stood up for themselves, in the end the general manager was to be the boss. The other officers and advisors, however dazzling, now needed sponsorship if they were to continue to twinkle:

DNS: Maureen's [CNA] influence is all directed at the HA. She's got an extraordinary amount of influence with them – but she wouldn't have got it without Gilbert's [DGM] backing.

'Let managers manage' was the first command of the new order. The initial priority was to establish control – only then could the new management begin. In some authorities, the old regime had been very rocky indeed:

DCh: [My] feelings [stemmed] from the very *odd* circumstances in which I became chairman. The previous chairman had wanted out. People were throwing bread pellets, knocking papers off tables in meetings. [Original emphasis]

A key part of the new order was therefore, to persuade, sideline or, if necessary, silence those who either could not or refused to take part in the new order. *In extremis*, and where it was held to be necessary, most people, with the exception of community physicians, could be removed. Thus, just as in some districts, people were retired as the new structures were created, so a potential threat still hung over those remaining senior staff whose performance was judged to be inadequate. Some argued that such powers had always existed but had never before been seized:

UGM: There's always been an opportunity to get rid of poor quality staff in the NHS but we've never taken advantage of it. We've walked away from the problems of poor staff and we need to face up to it.

Now, indeed, the problem was being faced, although the decision could be painful and long drawn out. Even new general managers who failed to come up to scratch could be removed:

DGM: I just couldn't get a paper on the unit structure from her [medical UGM] and she wouldn't discuss it with me . . . [Sacking her] was the toughest decision I've had to do. I didn't do it lightly. I had been concerned [for several months], so I started putting things in writing to her. She wasn't communicating and she wasn't getting information from the people in her unit. They didn't know what was going on . . . After fourteen months in the post we'd only had two papers from her and there was still no structure. The first structure [plan] came in June, the final deadline had been May and it wasn't a general management structure – and she herself hadn't written it anyway . . . I got someone in [a management consultant] to act as a facilitator to try and help improve communication . . . She was at loggerheads with all my directors . . . I kept telling her, 'Jane, it isn't working, you should speak to the chair', but she didn't.

Thus, the new leader of the team had the power to enforce a new organizational discipline. Leaders could also enforce a new organizational morality:

*DGM:* I think some people will never be satisfied and, if they are allowed to pursue things, the outcome will not be in the interests of the organization. At some point, you have to make a judgement and say, these are the ground rules, these are the reference points.

*DGM:* The trouble was, she started not telling the truth. I can accept someone who doesn't tell all the story slanting the issue – I might withhold something that's true – but telling downright lies I can't tolerate.

## Flexible staff, flexible structures

Teamwork thus took a new form. This major shift had several aspects. Not only was the new team directed but the new director had the chance to impose a much greater flexibility of membership and structure than had hitherto existed. Flexibility, indeed, was a watchword of the new management:

*DCh:* It [the NHS] is much more stagnant [than industry] – it's even worse than the NCB! . . . Of course, it's much more complex than the NCB . . . I've spent a lot of time explaining to people that management and administration are not the same thing. Administration is reactive; management is pro-active. It's a ghastly word but we have to use it. Management should always be thinking about the strategy. A very good example is the ambulance service pay structure . . . Our manager said that it was pretty awful – there were a number of Spanish customs to get rid of and a lot of overtime. He gave us two options. A was more expensive than B – but a lot more flexible. The instinctive reaction of the board was to go for B. I stressed A. I said we had to go for it. Now that's what I call *management* thinking. Quite rightly the treasurer resisted to the end and then caved in! [Original emphasis]

There were many kinds of flexibility in Griffiths. In the previous management arrangements, the DHSS laid down a national set of specifications for local organizational structure. It was DHSS which decided which posts were to exist in district health authorities, what their job specifications and titles were to be and which committees with what powers they were to sit on. Now, however, while there were still important central constraints, a much greater degree of freedom was permitted in local management arrangements. The new management team, for example, had a far more open membership. The old teams at region and district were exclusive affairs. DHSS had laid down just who could be a member and who could not. The new structure was more flexible. New trades and new advisors were welcomed on board:

*RPD:* Of course, personnel officers can now be members of the board and there's a lot more attention given to works . . . There is much more managerial interest in and control over the estate . . . The two neglected resources of the NHS – capital and people – have emerged as key things.

*RFD:* I'm probably chairing this meeting [a talk by a management consultant] because I'm currently paying for most of the management consultancy in the Western world!

[Just as membership of the local management team was more open, so too were the formal structures within which the team was to work. The new general managers had a chance to select both the team and the structures they wanted. The old bureaucratic rigidity imposed from Whitehall was to go:]

*ML (from the King's Fund):* We now have a marvellous opportunity to rid ourselves of the NHS's obsession with charts and boxes and to be flexible . . . good structures · do not drop out of the sky or get invented at the King's Fund!

*CNA:* Alex [DGM] isn't really into job descriptions. His style is, 'You're being paid. Get on with it. Tell me if there are any problems.'

*CNA:* Our formal structure is just for region! If Jimmy didn't have to submit a formal structure and lines of responsibility, I doubt if he would do. He's much more committed to getting a group of people together to solve things. He thinks structures are a form of pedantry – though they do satisfy the need to monitor and you can put a cost to structures. However, as soon as he's done that, I think he likes to depart from it, based on emerging needs. He sees one person as fitting several different roles over time. People are the resources, he thinks.

*DFD:* We've got this other apparatus, the district advisory group – or have we? Which doesn't meet. That's not a criticism. When it did meet it wasn't very productive . . . I believe it's got a meeting in a few weeks' time. I was quite astonished. 'Are you sure?' I said. My secretary convinced me. Well, I'll troll along and see what happens . . . It was probably seen by Jeff [DGM] as just an extension of DMT [the old district management team]. It's up to him.

The new flexibility extended not only to staff and to structure but to the roles that each team member filled. DGMs now had a wholly new opportunity to build powerful teams, regardless of members' original professional skills. If Sheila was excellent at detailed administration but weak on long-term vision, she could be placed accordingly. Jim, who had the opposite strengths, could fill in where Sheila could not, and vice versa.

*DGM:* Jean [DFD] did a super job, she created lots of new initiatives – though I have to say that she was not strong on implementation, she was an ideas woman . . . Tony [DMO] has picked up some initiatives on the quality side and he's done good things, though he's not good on the verbal side.

Here – so many argued – was a huge opportunity for the skilful general manager; a chance to cut the district's coat according to the cloth that was actually available:

*Asst UGM/DNS:* Professional background is immaterial, it's the ability to manage that counts. Management is about setting objectives and creating the right environment in which to achieve those objectives. It's all inherited – you can't acquire this ability – though you can improve on it.

*CNA:* Personalities are critically important in Griffiths and Jim [DGM] plays to personalities as no other structural arrangements could allow.

*DGM:* We've got to pick winners. We've picked three good people out of the woodwork at St Luke's. The [nursing] hierarchy stopped them in the past.

*DGM:* We're retaining a firm of accountants to oversee things [management budgeting], but I've given the job for handling this sort of thing to a pharmacist! A really super woman that I discovered.

Although Griffiths certainly imposed a structure of its own, it was, therefore, a framework with a very high degree of elasticity; of suppleness and pliability in the face of the storms, tides and eddies of change. This way, at least in theory, the service could respond with a much greater ease to the turbulence of its internal and external environment; to shifts in disease pattern, fluctuations in funding and the regular changes in personnel as staff retired, were promoted, or moved on to other jobs.

One consequence of such flexibility was the disappearance of any immediate equivalence between staff with the same title. In Wales, unlike England, each district had been obliged to appoint a chief nursing advisor at district level. Yet, just like many CNAs in England, most of their Welsh equivalents – CANOs – had been appointed to at least one other health authority task besides the provision of nursing advice. A key part of their formal position might differ, but in reality the new advisors' position was much the same in both countries. The old common role had gone and been replaced by a huge variety of jobs:

*CANO:* The cohesiveness in terms of common roles has gone in exactly the same way as it has gone in England because some do personnel, some do qualilty assurance, some do something else . . . And information previously that used to be sent simultaneously to all chief officers is now channelled personally and directly through DGMs, so there is an opportunity to be selective about how and to whom and what information is shared. All of a sudden, the CANOs have found that they are not party to the same amount of information at the same time – and that weakened the collective position, it weakens the professional position.
*INT:* How do you stand in relation to that?
*CANA:* I think I stand in the middle . . . One of my colleagues is very privy to the gems, these little treasures of information . . . We can sort of gauge our relationships on the level of, 'What day did you get that letter? Well, I've never seen it.'

The introduction of hybrid or joint posts affected chief nurses rather more than most other district managers. But this disappearance of a common, centrally prescribed role was fundamental to the whole of Griffiths. A breakdown of the traditional, rigid separation between one part of the service and another was crucial to the creation of an overarching general management. The managers and clinicians of tomorrow were to be crossbreeds, each ideally combining skills that up till now had been carefully segregated. The new type of organization was to have a new type of staff. Everyone was to be inter-disciplinary – doctors, nurses and accountants, too:

*DGM:* One of the great problems is the role culture – 'I'm a doctor', 'I'm a treasurer', 'I'm a nurse', etc. General management has to overcome this.

*CNA:* The previous DNO was very much an autocrat . . . and for her the district's nurses were always right. She was very much a tribalist. But lots of other people in the NHS want to care – treasurers and administrators and so on. It's not just nurses who care. I'm very sceptical of some modern nursing claims; the idea that we can claim monopoly rights on care.

*DFD:* The philosophy of finance here is to have very good liaison with other departments. We want to contribute to the whole. In other districts, accountants are seen as a very isolated profession commenting on other people's work – so we've advocated a multi-disciplinary approach . . . Too often finance departments are regarded as a law unto themselves . . . There are some treasurers who think their only role is to say no . . . [But] we need to know about how the NHS ticks. For me, there's a learning and a giving role. We need to know about the overall service and how it's run. I wouldn't expect to learn doctoring and nursing – just as I wouldn't expect them to learn accountancy – but we do need to know more about the services. Too often, we deal with expenditure for items that we don't have any clue as to what they're used for.

*DGM:* Everyone in the health authority needs some management training alongside their professional training. We're going to start management teaching for all the disciplines, based in the nursing school.
*INT:* Is this everyone except the doctors?
*DGM:* No! If they want management training, they will go through *my* system!

*DGM (and ex-doctor):* I tell the [new nurse] managers that the first eighteen months in the job is the worst because they will all have terrible paranoid conflicts between being a nurse and becoming a manager. The professional on one side of their head is saying different things to the businessman on the other side. I tell them that it's taken me a couple of years but they'll learn.

The new plan for the hybridization and cross-fertilization of all NHS staff was, of course, highly ambitious. None the less, many new managers felt there were real signs of some individuals breaking out of their old roles, of the new vision emerging:

*DGM:* The new UGM acute is a doctor by training – a paediatrician – but he doesn't want to be seen as a doctor. In fact he calls himself 'Mr'. He wants to be a DGM!

*CNA:* At a rough guess, at least two of [the DNSs appointed as new unit managers] have not changed their practice one bit and their managerial role is pretty well carried by the local administrator . . . They exercise a bit of oversight and all the rest of it, but they have remained primarily the matron or the senior nurse. About three of them have totally rejected their nursing role and function altogether – total abrogation – and it's a funny thing, the most interesting thing to watch is how people sign their letters. You can tell how they perceive themselves from the titles they use on their letters and – without getting too nitty gritty – for example, I wrote to Mrs Smith and I am most careful how I direct and address my letters. I wrote to Mrs Smith as supervisor of midwives asking her professional advice on a consultation paper relating to some aspect of the midwifery services. She sent back her response signed as a general manager. So I sent it back, saying, 'Please get this designation changed. I must have on record your advice as the supervisor of midwives' . . . I think she thinks I'm mad – this is sort of presented as 'silly bugger', you know . . . I'm trying very hard to get them to retain the acceptance of, the recognition of, a parallel, not a subordinate, but a parallel senior nurse role. And some of them are managing that tightrope, riding two bikes – you know that circus act of riding two bikes at the same time – very, very well indeed.

If some old areas of command – like the old DNO and DNS roles – were closed off in the new integrated structures, others now presented themselves. Whenever a gap in the market opened up, wherever there was an unfilled but important niche, a manager or advisor from a particular trade might potentially expand his or her range of activities. Anyone who had a comparative advantage over potential rivals for a task – whether in time, skill, effort, or the DGM's sponsorship – could move to fill that slot, sometimes in new and unpredicted ways:

*CNA:* The other thing I've realized is that the statistician needs a clinician to interpret what he's producing and I've actually spoken to the general manager and asked him, when he wants information for the health authority which is just data, would he please put it through me because, otherwise, we're not getting an actual clinical interpretation. We're just getting broad facts and if you know anything about the job, you could drive a coach and horses through it.

*DNE:* We've changed the structure of the nursing school completely since you were last here. We've become a department of education and staff development and we run management development courses which are for everybody, not just nurses – well, for everybody except doctors – but it does include all the paramedicals . . . We were being overwhelmed with non-nurses coming to us and saying, 'Could we come to you for development courses because nothing is being run for us?' About five years ago, long before the district personnel officer arrived, Charles [DGM] and I came up with this idea. But there's no conflict . . . The DPO is part of the district training forum, we're all part of the same team. We're merely taking things up, on an agreed basis, that the DPO can't handle. He's absolutely overwhelmed by privatization and manpower. He chairs our manpower group.

These last examples are drawn from the senior management team. But, since, in the future, all staff were to be hybrids, the abolition of many traditional ranks and roles had implications for the organization of every part of the service. All work was now to be arranged in wholly new ways; ways that were determined by a generalist's, not a specialist's perspective, by someone with a vision – so it was argued – of the whole, not the part. Everyone now had a new boss who could arrange work in the ways that he or she – not the individual trades – thought most fit. The long-term aim was to produce an entirely new type of integrated, inter-disciplinary organization. The following quotations cover nursing, medicine, portering, cleaning and local supplies:

*DGM:* The other bit I've been sorting out is the on-going discussion of how nurses will be managed by non-nurses. We've already decided that at the senior levels. The issue now is can sub-unit nurses be managed by non-nurses? I'm trying to stop the parallelism of the NHS tribes; to resource and train them and get clear support systems for a whole service.

*UGM (ex-doctor):* All I do is just see what people do. Health visitors are supposed to be generic – but in fact they spend 95 per cent of their time with children. So I see them as the nucleus of the new child health service. Again, district nurses are supposed to be generic – that's what they all say they are – but they spend 85 per cent of their time with the elderly. So I see them as the basis of the new service for the elderly.

*DGM:* We've now got nurses in management positions throughout the district – for example in theatre and outpatients. And in the long run we want doctors too. And in each area we want groups, teams to discuss utilization . . . We are working towards a new advisory structure in which there will be a corporate structure for a defined clinical area and others – apart from doctors – can legitimately join in the debate.

*UGM:* I felt the focus had to be the patient. Instead of professional groupings such as nursing I felt the grouping had to be clinical work. For example, trauma and orthopaedic services were given a manager . . . Overall, this has produced fifteen clinical services units . . . Given the importance of clinical decisions, I wanted doctors to take on a management role. They were cynical and reluctant . . . They compared it with Johns Hopkins. [Here] more work did *not* generate more money! However, I finally identified one consultant in each clinical grouping to take on a part-time clinical manager role – supported on a full-time basis by an assistant manager . . . I think the majority [of these] should be nurses but I don't believe that they all should be. [Original emphasis]

*Asst UGM/DNS:* I think my job will cover in-patient services such as domestics and linen. I'm very pleased about that. Things have gone full circle. These are the sorts of things that matrons used to control. The services suffered when domestics were split off. They will benefit from nursing control . . . [At the moment] we've got a nurse manager for nurses, a manager for the porters, a sterile supplies manager, a theatre assistant manager – but they're all going to come under the control of one manager. This must improve the service. The same is going to happen for A and E, for outpatients and night services. They'll be put together. I'm particularly anxious for the latter to happen. There's a great tendency in the health service to think that everything stops at five o'clock. I've got a senior nurse manager on duty after five, but she has no control over the porters and the clerks. There's also a registrar and an administrator in charge of beds. In the future, all this will be controlled by one person . . . [It needs to be because] no two managers think alike. You can spend half a day arguing . . . In the 74 reorganization the management tree mushroomed. There were so many managers that they never got their act together. You can't possibly decide what's best for the service, if every little group takes its own decisions.

Not everyone agreed. Though most of the managers to whom we spoke were enthusiastic supporters of the new vision, some were not. We have focused on the majority view, but there were some who, although critical of many of the old ways, still had their doubts about the new reforms on offer. To some ardent reformers of nursing, for example, Griffiths's emphasis on integration and hybridization seemed to threaten all that had so painfully been achieved in the previous two decades. Some nurse managers who had struggled to build a good nursing service now, so they argued, found all their efforts swept away:

> *Ex-CNO:* I do think that those of us who had found our way along a good path were suddenly mugged by Griffiths; knocked down, robbed and gave up.

> *CNA:* The DGM sees manpower planning for nursing as a function, not for nurses, but for personnel officers. Yes, nurses can have something to say about it, yes, they can give some advice about it – but manpower is personnel work . . . that's how he sees it and that's how the personnel director sees it.

> *RNO:* One of my support staff used to link very well with nursing personnel officers at district – that's almost entirely gone now. He tried to link with one a couple of months ago and there was an explosion. He was told he should have gone through the general manager. In the past, if I wanted to visit a hospital, I just used to ring up the DNO, now I have to ring up the UGM.

> *Acute DNS:* I can't say I welcomed having a UGM. The individual is fine. If I have to have one, he's as good as I'll get. But for the first time I'm responsible to a non-nurse and I have to put the case for things to an executive board – which irritates me. There's less freedom. We were very fortunate before. We had a good consensus team. And also, if I decided I wanted to do something, it was most unusual if Kathy [CNA] was unhappy about it. Whereas, now I have to explain everything to non-nurses and that takes longer and they may see things differently. I'm not sure if I ought to say this but I feel my job has lost in status. I'm not a person to put great weight on this. But before this I felt I was as much a leader as anyone else in the hospital – whether they were a consultant or the administrator. I feel now that I've been made more like the unit personnel officer. Instead of one of the directors, I feel like one of the support staff.

However, though it caused pain for some, for many other managers the new division of labour was both an opportunity for advancement and a chance for a much improved service. Omelettes could not be made without breaking a few eggs. Flexibility and integration were the ways of the future.

## Centralization – devolution

We have considered the new style of leadership and the new kind of team, the greater flexibility of structure and, lastly, the move towards hybrid staff despite the opposition it encountered from some managers. But there were other elements in Griffiths, too. Associated with all the ideas cited above, and overlapping with them – at least in part – was a major reorganization of the balance of devolution and central control. Part of the philosophy was outlined by a leading businessman at a conference for NHS managers:

> *BM:* You need as flat an organization as you can possibly get if you want change. You don't want twenty tiers. You need to be in touch with the troops. If something

has to go through several tiers, it gets filtered away. Once an organization is success-ful, you can afford more tiers – but as soon as things go wrong you need to flatten the organization again. You need to go straight to the root of things, to the people on the ground. In my company [a large clothing retailer] now, each marketing opportunity is a separate profit centre. Each is managed by a divisional board which is responsible for marketing, profit, etc. We at the centre provide them with dis-tribution, transport and so on – all the unimaginative things. All the creative things are done down there.

Similar devolution was being applied to the NHS. All kinds of matters were now to be pushed downwards at every level of the organization. One key move was to break district services down into just a few component parts or units – the acute hospital, community services and so forth – each of which had its own independent management structure which was supervised but not run by dis-trict. It was, ideally, up to local managers to devise the structures that suited their local circumstances, rather than these being imposed from the top (though each tier's plans for its new structure still needed approval from the tier above). The creation of units had begun in 1982 and was reinforced in 1984 with the arrival of general management:

> *DGM:* The health authority in 1982 had refused to devolve . . . So I decided that the best way forward was to identify centres of population around hospitals . . . We ended up with twelve locality managers in all . . . This proved very, very difficult to implement because . . . all the doctors and nurses, were up in arms . . . They'd heard it all before in 1974 and 1982 and nothing had happened then. You go round now!

> *DGM:* My attitude was that unit general managers could have whatever [unit] structure they liked, as long as they built in medical and nursing advice. I didn't care if they had ten little nigger boys – well, I might! I haven't been involved in any of the unit staff appointments – though I insisted they had the district personnel officer in as an assessor. But for the rest, I honestly didn't mind – unless they wanted my opinion . . . It's entirely up to the UGM as to how they do the financial administra-tion. In some places, it's been devolved to units with a senior post going there; in others, they're liaising with the district finance department.

> *Asst UGM/DNS:* The mental handicap unit will have its own accountant . . . They'll be here every day for half a day. It'll make a big difference. Information will be ready to hand. At the moment, we have to make a ten-mile journey or wait till they come out here. The other difference is that each of us will have an individual weekly meeting with the accountant so that they're on top of the situation – which is very important as it varies so much from day to day.

Devolution was not just from district to unit, it was also to be done within units – right down to individual consultants and ward sisters:

> *DFD:* Even when the DNSs held [nursing budgets at unit level], they didn't seem to me to be managing costs very actively. It probably needs more devolution to make sense because the numbers are too large.

> *DID:* More than a thousand patients [in orthopaedics] had been waiting for an operation for over a year . . . the average time for a 'non-urgent' hip replacement was four years . . . The waiting list . . . was held by an appointments clerk in an

office three hundred yards from the orthopaedics department. This distance created major problems – there was no contact. There was also no one to organize short-notice admissions or when the consultants went on leave. It was the orthopaedic surgeons who first noticed the problem, so we decided to provide them with some management support . . . We appointed a bed manager . . . with functional responsibility to the chairman of the orthopaedics department. They weren't part of records or nursing, nor what was then known as administration . . . This was crucial. They weren't seen as a management spy! . . . In the end we appointed an ex-orthopaedic medical secretary . . . and got her an office right in the middle of the orthopaedic wing. We had to remove a ward sister from her office to do this – which is not the work of a moment! . . . The bed manager was to attend ward rounds, to discuss ideas with doctors and nurses . . . to maintain the waiting list, to check bed availability day by day and to maintain staff rotas and holiday charts . . . Over a two-year period, the numbers on the list fell from 3,000 to 1,000 . . . The waiting time for a 'non-urgent' hip replacement is down to one year.

*CNA:* We've now got micros all over the hospital, every ward sister is to have one. Our policy is to give a whole lot of increased power to the ward sister. She is to be in charge of the budgets, the domestic staff, etc. We have very few DNSs. We want as much as possible to be given to the ward level. Very shortly we hope that the ward sister will be able to buy in services from the catering department.

However, if devolution was a crucial part of Griffiths, so too was an equal and opposite tendency. The movement of management towards the frontline was simultaneously coupled with a new type of central control. The two elements were closely connected. On the one hand, people were to be given much greater freedom and encouraged to be bold:

*CNA:* The [district] mission statement has really concentrated our minds. It says that . . . we don't, won't worry too much about local bureaucratic rules – if you can find a short cut, take it and we'll back you.

*DGM:* The question of taking risks is absolutely essential. In many organizations, not just the NHS, there's a tendency to keep your head down. But if we're going to achieve a change in culture, risks have got to be taken. Having weighed up the situation managers have got to be prepared to take risks.

But, on the other hand, the staff at lower tiers to whom so much had been devolved were now to be held responsible for the actions that they took:

*DGM:* General management enables people to go off and make decisions for themselves – as long as they accept accountability for those decisions.

*DGM:* I think that we are going from the old concept of a team to one of a lot of individuals acting on their own. In the past, everybody wanted to be involved but no one wanted to take responsibility.

Thus, staff were to go off and get on with it, but there were now targets to be met and their individual performance was to be monitored. The old pyramid in which a host of other trades served individual doctors was to be replaced by a new pyramid of central managerial control. Again there was a business model. NHS managers were advised in the following terms:

*BM:* Objectives need to be established by central management. If you don't clarify these, how can you expect your staff to know what they are? . . . An organization's task is to provide clear, achievable objectives. I can't comment on the right method for you, but in my company we rely on a mixture of meritocracy and hierarchy . . . We divide the group into various units. We delegate the profit objectives to divisional boards. Each management team's role is to implement the objectives – objectives decided by me and a small team. We design the mission, the vision – somebody has to do that . . . I call it flag planting. I'm always lifting it up and planting it several miles ahead of where we are. It's signposting – this is my job. I'm sure that's what's needed. Objectives are really the implementation of mission . . . We've found that hierarchy works far more efficiently than conferences. You get swifter decisions, easier communications and greater job satisfaction. If it seems unfair, it need not be.

This – or key elements of it – was the system now beginning to be applied to the NHS. One member of the NHS management board revealed the early plans at a conference:

*NHSBM:* The first key thing is the planning system . . . At the moment, we're looking at fourteen regional strategic plans. This is the first time it's been done intensively. We're judging the extent to which they meet national criteria and the management demands they'll make at region and district. We're also isolating what we consider to be the crunch points . . . The next major component is the review system. What have you done, is it what you said you'd do and, if not, why not? These meetings offer the chance for a major review both of strategic issues and issues of major topical concern . . . We have performance reviews of regions planned for February and March 1986. This will be a review of 1985. We have identified the crunch points and picked out the extremes of performance – indicators will give us an accurate measure of each region's performance . . . We've used PIs [performance indicators] for our review of the regions and we're asking regions to do the same for districts.

The same review system was to be applied at every level, not just to regions or districts or units but to individuals too; everyone was to face regular performance review:

*DCh (addressing a health authority meeting):* It is incumbent on us to make sure that our efficiency, our performance indicators, our throughput are all up to standard. Region didn't press us [during this last review] but they will [next year]. We need to make sure that we are as near the regional average as we can be.

*BM:* It's essential to review staff performance and provide individual incentives. I'm aware you're dedicated, otherwise you wouldn't be here today listening to a shopkeeper! But we need a variety of incentives, professional and financial. No one can be a success who works just for one of those. The majority of managers responsible for my company's success today are exactly the same as those who were managing it when it was failing ten years ago. How's it been done? We've told them the truth – we've stated our objectives. And we've monitored and recognized performance – as soon as a particular unit improved, we've rewarded everyone in it.

However, there were penalties as well as rewards in the new review system.

If performance was unsatisfactory, heads might roll. The new general managers were merely on three-year contracts, as some joked, a trifle nervously, when addressing management conferences:

*UGM:* As a UGM I have only 1,000 days to make my mark – but unlike Anne Boleyn, at least I know this from the outset!

*UGM:* I'll start with region. In our region we have the youngest RGM in the country. He would have been here today but his mother said (*loud laughter*) – I'm not worried about my contract (*laughter*).

So, although there was still the notion of a team, of working together, it was a radical shift from the old model. Teamwork now consisted in having a more global view and a wider range of skills; in being more oriented to the needs of the whole organization. But the new kind of team member was a more solitary being, no longer protected by union, profession or traditional hierarchy, but directly accountable to a manager through a system of personal review; a system that covered everyone and extended upwards to the chairman of the NHS management board. In some instances, very specific contracts with precise targets might be issued:

*DGM:* If we're going to get the message all the way down the line, we have to realize that there is a contract of management which probably didn't exist before. I have a contract with my UGMs and they have contracts with their line managers – we've agreed objectives, priorities and timing.

Moreover, because the devolved structure was to be closely monitored, devolution could be matched by very detailed intervention in those parts of the organization that general managers felt needed attention. Parts of the organization that the old administration had never reached could now find themselves subject to systematic central management intervention. Likewise, given their power to intervene at all levels, general managers could now subvert the traditional internal hierarchy within other disciplines, checking what was going on by gathering information from lower down and making new alliances there:

*Asst UGM (mental handicap):* There were no working relationships, no multi-disciplinarity [in this unit]. Everything was blamed on other people – on personnel or the administrators. No one ever took responsibility. The unit got quite severely reprimanded by district . . . The old DNS took early retirement, I got the development job, the deputy administrator was withdrawn. James [DGM] and his deputy actually came to all our UGM meetings – one or other of them – and they set us objectives. They didn't pull any punches.

*DGM:* I actually wrote the bulk of the constitution [of the nursing and midwifery professional advisory group]. There was a lot of nonsense about having just DNSs. I said no – it must represent the bulk of nurses. In fact, we ended up with a compromise. We needed a very good chair so in fact that appointment is not elected. Hopeless if it was. We might get a staff nurse. The previous chair was elected – a sweet and good member but hopeless as a chair, she babbled endlessly. So I appointed John.

*DGM:* Where I'm getting real support is from nurses in middle management . . . I'm getting real support from them *against* the senior nurse managers. I'm really surprised, but it's true. [Original emphasis]

## Computerized information

The new central monitoring was not just a matter of structure, reports and political information – crucial although all these might be. At its very heart lay the development of new methods of generating routine numerical data on performance, and the systematic use of the information systems that already existed but which hitherto had never played any serious role in detailed management. It was here, along with leadership, that the old clinical management had failed. Community physicians had lacked the power to use the data. Nurse managers had not known how to. No one else had access to clinicians. Now, however, the new management was to reach deep into the heart of the service. General management's grasp was to be based on systematic, quantitative information on all the key aspects of the daily work of the NHS:

*NHSBM:* We want a circumstance where information is not a funny thing that you put on a funny form because a funny man from the NHS management board asked you for it. We want a climate where the general manager is actually beating on the information director's door saying, 'For Pete's sake, tell me what happened last week' . . . Information is the lifeblood of our management system.

Again, the ideal model was the private sector. One regional manager looked longingly to the management information systems he had encountered in the firm run by the architect of the NHS reorganization:

*RGM:* I went to see Roy Griffiths in his office at Sainsbury's and while I was talking to him, his secretary handed him a piece of paper. He looked at it and said, 'OK'. I asked him, 'What do you mean, "OK"?' and he said, 'My organization is OK today'. It turned out he had just six measures on that piece of paper and from those he could tell what the state of Sainsbury's health had been the day before; things like the amount of money taken yesterday, the freshness quotient – the amount of stuff still on the shelves – the proportion of staff on duty, and so on.

Equivalent measures, if they were to come about in the NHS, were possible only through the use of modern technology. The new balance of devolution and central control was heavily dependent on microprocessors. New, computer-based methods simultaneously offered the possibility of affecting both local and central practice and were being developed in all parts of the service; particularly so in the finance departments:

*DFD:* When I went to X district [twenty years ago] control at unit level was almost entirely absent. We used to send them monthly budget statements, but they were very summary – and they had to be because of the technology of accounting. It was partly manual extraction . . . Changes in technology have facilitated far more active financial management.

*DFD:* We now have pharmacy and X-ray department information on line for the last fortnight. It's drugs and disposables where the costs are out of control – it's here where we're going to get reamed . . . Right now, we just spend and we don't know what's going on. When I ask, I just get wringing of hands and rolling of eyeballs . . . This sort of information will make a huge difference to health authority meetings!

## Conclusion

The new management was, therefore, based on a wholly new set of principles: on systematic monitoring, on a single line of command, on an integrated structure, on the rule of generalists not specialists, on greater devolution as well as greater central control, on flexible staff and flexible structures, on hybrid staff members who would know something of everyone's job, on micro- as well as macro-management. Such changes, in turn, facilitated a new role for the new boss. Once the new structures had been put in place, once there was a smooth flow of precise and crucial information to the centre, once every individual within the organization had taken on a greater personal responsibility – and a responsibility for the whole and not just the part – then the general manager could sit back a little. Radical devolution, when coupled with modern information systems and regular review, gave potential scope for a new, more strategic role for senior management:

*DGM:* [In] the old system . . . there were very few management stops so that everything floated to the top . . . We were just fire fighting, reactive not pro-active . . . I'm trying to pull senior managers back from the day to day issues, to get them to think about things two or three years from now, about the management of change issues . . . Management has always got to be at one role back.

*DGM:* Last year the RCN were playing merry hell with me! And all the professions had their professional bodies getting at me – but I carried on! Now I can just sit back! (*pause*) I do sit back. My job is to lead the orchestra – I have a devolved style of management – to deal with the tone and pitch of things. It took me two years of bloody hard work to get here and I'm enjoying it now. I don't have to play every instrument, but I know the score.

So the new structures and the new style of teamwork could free the general manager to think about the big issues; or so it was argued. In the next chapter, we examine the methods being developed for the biggest issues of all – the drive to improve both the cost and the quality of the service.

The last chapter considered the new philosophy of pro-active management rather than humble administration. It focused on the way general managers – and staff who had joined the crusade – applied the new model to the NHS. This chapter examines two further fundamental aspects of the creed: the simultaneous managerial emphasis on quality and on cost. Getting value for money had two key stages: first, examining how money was spent and the quality of service produced by that spending; then considering how it might be spent more effectively. Every aspect of the service needed to be considered: transport, maintenance, supplies, laundry, the division of labour between different types of staff, the way patients were actually treated, the cost and quality of different types of care, the systems for providing financial and clinical advice.

The drive for lower costs and increased quality was conducted in very different ways in different regions, districts and units. Although the DHSS provided a lead, a good deal was left to the tiers below. How things were actually done, therefore, depended a good deal on the varying skills, interests and circumstances of the new management teams. However, although the details varied, overall there could be no doubt that this radical revision of the NHS entailed a major diminution of clinical power; a reduction not just of the power of individual clinicians but also of their professional associations. Cost and quality were no longer matters to be left wholly to the decisions of particular trades. General managers wanted specialist advice, not specialist control.

## Value for money

Of all the many aspects of Griffiths, it was cost reduction that was at its very heart. Just as the new emphasis on teamwork and personal assessment meant the rise of personnel managers, so the stress on efficiency and active cost management meant that treasurers were to be turned into finance directors. The emphasis on detailed costing was new to the NHS, as one CNA recalled:

> CNA: Up till 76, money wasn't an issue. If you spent more than you were allocated you got your fingers rapped, but you were still allocated more! . . . Then cash limits

came in. Before that DNOs didn't know how many nurses they could afford . . . The statistics we sent to the Department were worse than useless.

The efficiency drive had many aspects. Some got more public attention than others, but every part of the service became the subject of financial scrutiny. Competitive tendering for hospital catering and cleaning was the most famous, or infamous, part of the efficiency drive, striking as it did at the very lowest paid workers in the service. It was not met with great enthusiasm by most managers; indeed, it was largely forced on authorities by national politicians. None the less, it had been done and some savings had been made:

*DGM:* We've also privatized hotel services [e.g. catering]. Every contract has gone in house but we've saved £140,000 through doing this.

Rationalizing the distribution of the district hospital system had a great deal more appeal to managers (if not always to local residents). Many districts had a patchwork of institutions built in several different eras and costing a good deal to maintain. Locating services on a common site could potentially save a good deal of money. It was now felt by many clinical staff and managers that patients had in the past been kept in hospital for unnecessary lengths of time. Beds could, therefore, be closed while still keeping – or even increasing – the throughput of patients. Reducing the length of stay was therefore at the heart of the search for lower costs:

*CNA:* Acute services were spread over three sites here, separated by two main roads . . . It was a major contribution to our expenses . . . In the process [of rationalization] we've had to shed several hundred beds – that's mostly completed now. Beds of all kinds have gone – nothing's been sacrosanct . . . We haven't reduced the clinics but we've cut beds and wards. We've reduced the estate and we're making what's left work harder. We have targets for bed utilization and the district is on target. Our consultants had got into pretty sloppy ways of working.

Other aspects of the service were also being closely examined. Indeed, radical managers saw opportunities for cost improvement in every nook and cranny:

*RCh:* The greatest task for management in the NHS today is inventory control. This is where business and the NHS are furthest apart . . . We have £20 million tied up in stock. We're building a regional distribution centre for two and a half million pounds – as many other regions are. If we can't get our inventory down to £15–16 million, I shall be very surprised.

*DGM:* We're dieselizing the ambulances which will save on fuel . . . At the moment, we've got management consultants looking at the laundry. It's very good dealing with them as they're trying to break into the market, so they are only charging a percentage of the savings and not a fixed fee. I'm also negotiating with the Council to see if we can take over all their laundry and also provide the meals on wheels and the day centre transport. In return we would let them do reprographics and share transport with them. Because we're all sharing this huge county every day and all these cars and vans are passing each other – it's ridiculous.

*UGM/DDQ/CNA:* An orthopaedics consultant is probably the one outstanding manager in the district at the consultant level. In four hours, the two of us saved £90,000 ranging from toilet rolls to catheters. We advertised the post of management resources officer on the basis that the incumbent would have to save £100,000 per year every year or the contract would cease. We appointed an outstanding nurse who has saved us over a million pounds in his first year – so he's secured his job for the next ten years!

## Skill mix

Since health care is a labour-intensive industry, most NHS money went on wages. Not only were manpower and womanpower costly, they were becoming more so with demographic change. In some districts, for example, nursing was badly affected by an acute and growing shortage of staff:

> *CNA:* In comparison with the inner London hospitals running at 20 and 25 per cent [nursing] vacancy factor, we're running at 15 per cent. So we are a damn sight better than Hammersmith and Paddington. But it is not good because 15 per cent is worse than last year when it was in single figures. The trend is rising.

> *CNA:* We are very low on staff [in the mental handicap hospital] . . . a 24-bedded ward might have three or four nurses on during the day. It's not enough; not to do the things that modern care of the mentally handicapped requires – which is more than just personal hygiene. There's the education and teaching them to be members of society and so on.

Since labour was expensive and in short supply, the solution to the problem, so managers urged, was to reorganize the way it was used. Value for money meant a much more efficient allocation of tasks, a huge drive for a new division of work among the labour force. How should this be done? The issue was too important to be left to the trades. Under the old system, every trade had a say in its division of labour. Though some were far more powerful than others, the allocation of tasks had been negotiated between trades and not according to some master plan. Inside the rough boundaries that emerged from this negotiation, trades tried to run their own work according to their own traditions and evolving interests. Detribalization meant, therefore, not just a new type of teamwork but a huge reduction of occupational power. The professional and trade union bodies which had patrolled the old division of labour were now to be demoted. Those who had fought against militant unions in the 1970s now, in the 1980s, turned their sights on the professions:

> *DPO:* My best experience was at region . . . one of the things I was responsible for was the ambulance service. They were very tough and militant. I always felt I'd seen the very toughest – unless I'd been in Liverpool. This was the time in the late seventies when the unions were fairly gung-ho. It was pre-Maggie. In that job – which was supposed to have a regional perspective – I was spending up to 75 per cent of my time on the ambulance service. We went at it very intensively for two years – but we cracked it. It's still my major achievement. The biggest thing in my career. We actually got management back on the job.

*DGM:* The doctors, in terms of conservatism, are at the extreme end of the spectrum. It's the trade unions that have felt the Thatcher government most. But there's not much difference between the professions and the trade unions. The BMA is just the most successful trade union of them all.

### Nursing skill mix

Our examples of the drive to get management in charge of the division of labour are taken from nursing, much the largest user of health service labour and a key target for the new chief executives. To understand the battle that ensued, some attention must be given to the internal reform movement that currently existed within nursing. Since nurses had increasingly managed their own affairs before Griffiths, its professional leaders had begun to develop new ways of organizing their work. Many nurses realized that the old ways needed serious modification. What the new managers feared, however, was that the schemes favoured by the trade itself were the product of professional self-interest and an inadequate scientific training. There was, then, a sharp difference in outlook between those nurses who looked for professional solutions and those who had become general managers.

The staffing solutions proposed by the professionalizing nursing elite which dominated much of the RCN and the academic side of nursing involved two main arguments. Patients, it was held, needed far more individual attention; attention best given by a much more highly trained staff. This more professional workforce, although considerably more expensive and a lot smaller in numbers, would be so much more effective that it could substitute for the traditional, vast, ill-educated nursing labour force. Some of the more junior ranks of nursing could therefore be abolished and were, indeed, already being frozen out:

*DNS:* The role of auxiliary nurses . . . came up at the last HA meeting. A Labour member wanted to make sure that we weren't sacking any auxiliaries. We're not but we're not recruiting any. When vacancies occur we're converting to trained nurses . . . I would hope that we don't have to recruit more auxiliaries in the future.

Other managers were sceptical. Nursing, so they argued, was necessarily labour intensive and much of the work required only a low level of skill:

*Asst UGM/DNS:* The CNA came round one of the wards because there'd been a lot of complaints from patients and pressure sores were going up – we've got a very low level of staffing. She said that in the future maybe we'd need fewer staff – but that they would be much better trained and more adaptable, 'Wouldn't that be best?' I said, 'Fine, but four nurses can't do the work of six'. It's the nature of the work. We need lots of pairs of hands when we're dealing with very dependent patients.

There were equally grave managerial doubts about some of the new modes of work organization that had enthused so many in the trade. The 'nursing process', for example, was a system which had recently swept across the service. In this method, each patient's nursing needs were catered for through careful individual assessment, planning, treatment and treatment evaluation. Here was a bold step forward; one which the accrediting bodies – in England the ENB – had insisted on as a prerequisite of professional training. But did this complex programme actually work? Some managers had their doubts:

> *Deputy DGM/CNA:* The nursing process has had an extremely disturbing effect. It's been under-rated in its complexity and over-rated in its productivity. Above all it's never been evaluated. Like most things in nursing, it's been put in *ad hoc*. There's never been any parallel system of evaluation.

Given these and other doubts about the new professional model of nursing, many managers looked instead to very different solutions. Could some jobs be done just as well by less qualified staff? Might other jobs be done better by very different trades? And did some jobs really exist – might there not be surpluses in some areas as well as shortages? Many different areas of the service might need to be reorganized:

> *HSR:* I've been producing information about the staffing ratios in mental hospitals. The range is threefold. Input doesn't guarantee output, but we do need to tackle the variations . . . The staffing ratios in many mental hospitals have been the same for many years – some possibly for a hundred years!

> *Asst UGM/DNS:* I want to look at night duty seriously. It causes apoplexy among the night sisters when I mention this. We've got sisters on every floor. Do we need this? When I walk around at night half of them are not there. So there's too much hierarchy. It's terribly sensitive because they all earn far more money than on days – 30 per cent more. Are we getting value for money here?

> *DDQ/DMO:* We've just done some work on our health visiting service for the elderly. We have a special service with nearly twenty 'autonomous professionals' which costs over £200,000 a year. I got a very good woman, a sociologist, to do an observational study of 800 visits. Only 23 of them were concerned with post-medical care. Most of them were basically social work visits – yet they'd had no social work training and didn't know about all the relevant services, pension rights and so forth. So what were they doing?

The old division of labour was tied more to the interests of the trade than to those of the client. As we shall now see, this led, so many new managers argued, to an unusual and damaging perspective upon clients.

## Customer service

If VFM (value for money) and a more efficient skill mix were central creeds in the new model of management, so also was a new vision of the client. Clients too were to be viewed in financial terms. They were no longer to be seen as patients – that was the old medical and nursing model – but as customers. Of course, managers recognized that there was and always had been a powerful movement within health care to treat patients with greater courtesy and to respect their rights as human beings. But from the business perspective, this focused too much on the supply side and not enough on the demand:

*DCh:* We all pay for the service – £292 per annum. For that amount of money we ought to get a very good service.

*HSR:* Isn't the key thing to overcome the fact that the medical profession, with a very strong tradition of paternalism, is not used to seeing patients as customers?

*MC:* Are people treated like individuals? Are their needs respected? Why should the NHS worry about this? If you think about commercial organizations, it's obvious why they need to do this – they're in a competitive environment. *In Search of Excellence* is a book we all turn to.[1]

Not only did customers pay for the service, they were now on the brink of revolt against the way they were conventionally treated; or so argued one of the most popular speakers on the management lecture circuit:

*HSR:* We have some very dissatisfied customers – and, of course, we have some dead ones! . . . Up till now, the consumers have been very quiet but I think it's all going to change. People just aren't going to be tolerant any longer . . . I'm sorry to be the fellow to spoil the party.

General managers, therefore, had a central role to play in stimulating their staff to treat clients as customers rather than patients: records were to be checked, service contracts established:

*DDQ/Deputy DGM:* We need to set standards of service, e.g. to say to radiographers, 'What's a fair period of time between you taking the X-ray and the results being back not just to the consultant but to the patient?' Another thing that we're thinking of at the moment is taking a sample of one in a hundred records and seeing if we can examine the quality of feedback to the individual patient.

But it was not sufficient just to set standards and check records. If customer service was to get the priority it deserved, managers needed to get out of the office and see for themselves what was happening in the wards and waiting areas. MBWA (management by walking about) was a fundamental part of the new order. Some of the new leaders made tours of inspection and told others to do likewise:

*RGM:* I increasingly sit in outpatients and just watch. I've also invited members of the professional staff to do the same. The last time I was in a hospital, the WVS shop was shut, the clerks were talking among themselves, the gents' toilet was filthy – and all the locks were off the doors. When I visit a hospital these days, I always go in the visitors' toilets. Not many staff do that. And I can assure you that not many of my managers are going to get productivity bonuses on the basis of the state of the visitors' toilets! There was an old lady sitting in the corner who'd clearly been forgotten. We then went into a ward – superb clinical care but I have to say that the patient environment is not what I would want. The ward sister was not on duty – this may be grossly unfair but I've never seen a ward sister on duty in the last three years. There was a lovely colour telly – a lovely big job – but on top of it there was a small black and white set. I checked and the set hadn't worked for months and months. The sister put chitties in and nothing happened. I blame the sister and the managers of the hospital. There was a lovely day-room but it was locked because the picture window was broken last week. They'd put the chitty in and nothing had happened. This is unacceptable . . . How often does your hospital offer patients a choice of times as to when they can come in and say, 'Which would be convenient for you?' It doesn't require money but it does require that the patients' time is important . . . How many of you have been in your antenatal clinics recently? I have to tell you they are abysmal. Women are treated like cattle. How many of you have listened to patients who've been to A and E recently? It's OK if you're seriously ill – superb treatment. But if you take a child with a broken ankle – well! All it needs is words – a bit of explanation.

Monitoring, therefore, was seen as crucial to good customer service and could be done both formally and informally. But monitoring by itself was not enough. It had to be combined with intensive training in the new culture. Given their previous attitude, staff had to be taught how to treat clients as customers. Again, there was a private sector model:

*MC:* When British Airways developed their training programmes, they put every-one in together. I'd like to see doctors in with nurses and porters on the same course.

*RGM:* We had British Airways managers up to talk to us recently – they're compet-ing with other airlines and they've all got the same costs. What makes people fly Singapore Airlines is the quality of the treatment they get from the cabin staff. So at BA everyone of their 40,000 staff – from the pilots down – went through a customer sensitization programme. Of course, we're talking about half a million staff in the NHS, but that shouldn't deter us.

## The quality of care

Customer service has several possible meanings. So far we have focused pri-marily on the drive for spruce porters, clean toilets and doctors who consider the patients' time as well as their own. But the drive for quality touched on every aspect of the NHS. If money was being wasted on unnecessary stock or inefficient transport, then there was that much less to go on patient care. If expensive staff were allocated to jobs which cheaper staff might perform equally well then, again, the needs of other customers suffered. The quality of care was therefore of central concern in the new general management doctrine. Before Griffiths, the quality of care had been left mainly to the professional carers. Administrators simply paid the bills, handled the paperwork and supplied the buildings and equipment. In the theory of general management, however, the new executives took a far more active interest in the product. At the same time, the new system would work only if clinicians too were actively involved:

*UGM/DDQ/CNA:* Quality can be maintained under a cost-cutting system only when professionals play an active part in setting standards and monitoring. The key question is not pounds, shillings and pence, but the quality of care for pounds, shillings and pence.

At the core of the new strategy was an emphasis upon better information about the distribution, cost and quality of routine clinical practice. Such infor-mation was not just for managers alone. Of course it permitted centralized monitoring, as we noted in the last chapter, but it also permitted, it was hoped, clinicians to take a radically different approach to their own practice. Only they could interpret certain key aspects of the data and only they could exert systematic clinical pressure on each other. Routine information about the cost, load and quality of their practice would enable each clinician to plan his or her own work with an effectiveness and efficiency that had hitherto been impossible.

If every clinician were simultaneously supplied with details of their fellow team members' practice, this might break down the old insularity and individualism, creating, for the first time, common standards and a new set of problems for joint enquiry. Such data, since they dealt with individual performance were, of course, highly sensitive and clinicians needed time to get used to the idea. They nevertheless provided a radically new basis for negotiation. The new clinical team could now make plans in which everyone's actions were far more coordinated than had ever been possible before. And where peer pressure failed to do the trick, the general manager could, so it was argued, help out, suggesting areas that needed urgent consideration. A great variety of new information systems in medicine, finance and nursing were therefore under urgent consideration. And even where there were no new technical systems, managers were beginning to insist that clinicians had a duty to think far more broadly than ever before about their work and its organizational consequences; to make careful plans in consultation with their colleagues and the managers of the unit and district. Doctors, above all, were the target:

> *DGM:* What happens with information systems is that they open up doctors to peer pressure, e.g. about the length of stay or about their expenditure on drugs. This will happen when the information systems go in over the next year and a half . . . Standards can be set within a range and the staff set them for themselves. When they have feedback from us in how far they've gone towards achieving those standards, then they have the information to carry the discussion further . . . The new-style management is not about bringing clinicians to heel. Instead, it's about making them grow up. It's about making them take responsibility for doing things which they know in their hearts are right.

> *DFD:* My view is that we've got to develop an information system which can actually tell consultants what they're spending. Right now we haven't a clue what activity is going on. We don't want arbitrary cuts, but we do want a costing of their activity. Once we've got this then we can start probing . . . Then we can say, 'Mr X spent £50,000 on drugs last month; Mr Y, with the same case mix, £100,000'. Then I'll say to the UGM, 'You have a problem here . . . You need a policy.'

The new policy for managing clinicians could be implemented in many different ways and each district tried a different mix of initiatives: some went for discussions with individual doctors, some hoped that pressure from colleagues would win the day, some had brought in management consultants, some had involved health authority members. Even nursing information systems might also provide useful information on medical practice:

> *DGM:* We are starting to involve doctors in the management process – by talking to

them, by not just going for the medical advisory committee but going for corridor conversations, trying to get individual views.

*DDQ/CNA:* The doctors have been very responsive to the clinical budget findings. These are being kept fairly close to the management consultants which I think is reasonable because it is still a sensitive area. I mean they are looking at cost per in-patient day and they are making changes among themselves, so as a peer group I think they are doing a bit towards that.

*DGM:* I hope the doctors will be OK. They've been held accountable as a corporate lump. We hope that group pressure will do the trick. I'm not going to argue the toss with them. I'm not qualified to do that – but they are. They've got to put pressure on each other. Tied in with all this is the American system of peer review. We have to get that going here.

*DFD:* I told him [consultant cardiologist] 'Shirley [DGM] will want a plan for clinical services'. 'What's that? We just fit pacemakers when we need them.' 'No', I said, 'We want a plan. What are your criteria? How many are likely to be needed in the district's population? And we want some calculation of their opportunity cost' [i.e. what might be done with the money if the cardiologists spent it in other ways]. Shirley wants all the clinicians to analyse their activities – and then control them, which is the bit they're not terribly keen on!

*DDQ:* I've been very pleased with the way I've managed to get the health authority's quality panel to look at the PIs [performance indicators] for each medical specialism . . . It's a good way into medicine . . . My technique is to send the PIs to a [medical] division and then invite one or two consultants to a meeting of the panel. It's very, very fruitful. It's a two-way thing. The last one we did was the urologist. We thanked him and he said that it had been very helpful as he hadn't looked at the figures before . . . When we send out the PIs we now produce a comment by a UGM because even the clinicians aren't always used to analysing statistical information.

*DFD:* Monitor . . . is a nursing quality and nurse-planning tool . . . but what I want from it . . . for proper costings . . . are the levels of patient dependency . . . Without proper costings, doctors have no control. Doctors need to know what is being spent . . . It makes no sense just to have bed numbers . . . If I have a mixed specialty ward, e.g. the Jones ward which is mixed radiotherapy and haematology, I need to have a dependency figure for the haematology patients – say 42 per cent – bang! Like that!

Getting doctors to think about their own and others' work was a delicate business. Sometimes, the new managers spoke out firmly and one or two even acted that way, on occasion:

*DGM:* It's no good doctors treating me as if I've got an American Express card. We need to be able to say, 'I'll tell you what I've got in resource allocation and I'll tell you what I want in terms of performance'.

*DGM:* Doctors are either going to have to accept line management responsibility or else be locked out of the information systems. Clinical freedom is diminishing all the time.

*DFD:* Jill [DGM] takes them on full frontal. There's a stunned silence at medical committees! I'm not sure she recognizes this herself . . . She does things that are outrageous in an NHS context. Still they need shaking up . . . Her attitude is refreshing. She challenges unchallengeable things.

Caution, however, was the more normal approach to medical individualism. Doctors had to be picked off one by one. The central strategy in developing a more corporate medical approach was to work with those medical staff who were friendly and bide one's time with the rest:

DDQ: When I say I work by stealth, I mean that I've come to the conclusion that the only way to work with doctors is to work with one or two who are interested and hope that the rest join in – you can't proselytize or bleat about care . . . My philosophy is to work with the good and ignore the bad – and then eventually the bad will realize that they are missing something and want to be involved.

DGM: Clinical budgeting will be approached in different ways in different districts. You can't force it. You have to find friendly consultants. Budgeting can't lead management – it's entirely the wrong way round.

DGM: My target is the younger doctors. It's a waste of time working with the older generation.

As these quotations suggest, such strategies did not work with every doctor. But, even with the obstinate, the general manager could still hope that the wheel of fortune might one day tip the recalcitrant clinician direct into the killing grounds:

DGM: You have to pick them off one by one . . . For example, we've got a very difficult surgeon here. We've been wanting region to discipline him for eighteen months. He refuses to discuss anything with us at all. But he does want new equipment. I said to him, 'Fine. There's just one small thing. You'll have to sit down and discuss your workload with me. It won't be contractually binding, but we have to discuss it.' And, you know, within two days he did it! Yet before this he'd refused to see me.

## Active nursing management

Since nursing was less of a priority than medicine, the time and resources devoted to nursing information systems in the NHS were on a far smaller scale. However, the clinical budgeting systems developed for doctors could be used by nurses too. At the same time, nurses in some districts were beginning to use more sophisticated methods for measuring workload and quality such as Criteria for Care and Monitor (most of the examples given below are taken from one district which was a pioneer in these matters). As with doctors, the introduction of clinical information systems had to be undertaken with caution. All clinicians had been trained to think of care, not cost, and none were used to having their performance compared:

RNO: It [clinical budgeting] has been sold to the nurses there as a new way of organizing care, not as a new way of organizing resources. And that's absolutely essential. Given the way nurses are trained, they'd never accept it if it was sold to them in purely financial terms. They're trained to think in terms of care . . . So it's absolutely fundamental that clinical budgeting is not presented in terms of efficiency savings. They'll never accept it in those terms.

And again, as with doctors, the aim of the new information systems was to get the clinical staff themselves to analyse their own performance and to learn collectively from their peers:

*Asst UGM/DNS:* No one [is] saying, 'You shall [or] you shan't do this or that' . . . The individual wards [only] know their own [scores] . . . [But, through Criteria for Care and Monitor] nurses could actually see on the graph where their time was going and it helped us to identify so clearly for the first time how much time was actually being spent on patient care, how much time was being spent on clerical and other duties . . . I think the staff have realized that certain wards were coming out of the study extremely well and it appeared to be down to organization within the ward by the ward sister . . . it was a case of here very clearly and very objectively one ward in the same hospital with the people you know, your colleagues, your peers – some colleagues are achieving certain things, [while] someone in the ward next door with the same levels of staff and approximately the same workload is not . . . Why? . . . It has made us see that you have first got to do something about all these other aspects before you start putting in any more resources. You just don't go on adding staff to a situation that is really being mismanaged. You try and get your internal organization right and then you put in what you need when it is more clearly identifiable.

However, developing a more active approach to clinical nurse management involved more than new information systems. If managers needed to place serious limits on medical individualism, the problem with some nurses lay, so it was argued, in their extreme sense of hierarchy. The new system demanded a greater, not lesser, sense of freedom from nurses; a willingness to speak out in a way many had never done before:

*DGM:* The key thing that has happened this year is that the senior nurses in the advisory group are really beginning to work as a team and they're starting to have confidence in themselves – so much so that they now have sufficient confidence to disagree with us and with each other. This is an incredibly healthy sign.

The new information systems and the change in attitudes created two further possibilities. The first was of peer pressure being exerted, not just within a trade, but between clinical trades. Information systems were at the heart of the new multi-disciplinary style of teamwork:

*DGM:* [Due to management budgeting] I think we will be able to allow the nurse, the ward sister to manage that budget and I think we will have consultants putting pressure on nurses to actually provide a more effective service.

*Asst UGM/DNS:* The consultants we've got here – I've only had to confront one in a dramatic sort of way, but at the same time I offered him a sort of carrot saying, 'Look, OK, I've got to say, "No". You can't admit any more patients to that particular ward because of the pressure you're putting them under.' I did have the backing of the fact that we had got our statistics on workload which was a wonderful weapon. But at the same time as I was saying, 'No more patients, we can't cope', I was saying to him, 'Can we please get together and look at the types of patient you are admitting and what you are trying to achieve and see whether or not our resources can be used more effectively to help your patients, rather than you just throwing them in at us and us not really knowing what we are trying to do'.

The second possibility created by the new information systems was a wholly different position for nursing within health care – or at least for a management elite among nurses:

DDQ/CNA: In my opinion, nursing has an unprecedented opportunity under Griffiths to gain its portfolio . . . We need to provide a measure by which we test performance daily, weekly, monthly, yearly.

DDQ/CNA: 40 per cent of the district is now evaluated by Monitor . . . It's given us a mighty strong voice locally . . . in actual fact . . . Brian [a doctor and chair of the medical advisory committee] has been worried recently because part of the Infirmary has been measured and part has not and there is a tendency now for the authority to say, 'Oh, but we have measurement there, so we have to go for that one' . . . It's an extremely powerful, potent, political weapon.

This managerial approach to the reconstruction of nursing was very different from the professional model of reform discussed earlier. In that other model, the way forward for the trade was to model itself upon the egalitarian traditions of medicine and build a community of peers from the total body of nurses through the creation of a smaller but more highly trained workforce. By contrast, those who backed general management felt that nursing would always require many pairs of hands. Their vision of the future was that of a clinical elite at the ward sister level. Here and here alone could a body of real professionals be created. This clinical elite would be sharply separate from the massed ranks of nurses who performed the more humdrum nursing duties. Their task, instead, would be to allocate, monitor and evaluate the rest of the nursing labour force on a truly scientific basis. This, so it was argued, was the only way to create an efficient and effective nursing service. Here, also, lay the only possibility of creating nurses who could work as equals with doctors in the new, integrated health care teams.

## Managerial advice, professional advice

The corporate approach to quality and cost constituted a fundamental break with the syndicalist approach to the organization of health care. There was a new business model of the client, of the peer group, of the division of labour and of clinical performance. The new general managers circumvented the old administrative and advisory structures through which the specialist trades had been organized and challenged their right to organize themselves in the way they thought fit. It was now the prime duty of general managers, not of the clinical trades, to form the overall climate and particular mechanisms through which the new approach to the cost and quality of care might best be created:

> *DGM:* It's my responsibility to promote the environment where this sort of activity can take place . . . [And] it's the general manager responsible for a particular clinical area who has the task of discussing with the clinicians in that area what are reasonable standards for them to set.

But if the duties of general managers were clear enough, certain problems still remained. General managers might know how to manage, but did they have sufficient expertise for the massive task of restructuring clinical care? Three sorts of knowledge were needed: technical knowledge about clinical care and its evaluation; cultural knowledge of the outlook, vocabulary and intimate rituals both of management and of the clinical trades, so that the two sides could communicate easily; and political knowledge – how the service was actually run, which clinicians held real power, how they might best be approached. The dilemma of clinical expertise was tackled in different ways according to local dispositions and circumstances. One obvious solution was to appoint an ex-clinician as general manager:

> *DGM (ex-administrator):* I say that a nurse who becomes a good general manager will be a better general manager than me because I've not got operational knowledge of the service. The key issues are understanding the psychology of doctors and the real needs of the patients. Any general manager who's been involved in the delivery of care has a real advantage. It's really helpful if you've been a nurse or a doctor.
>
> *DGM (ex-doctor):* It's been very important in enabling me to manage the district that I'm both a clinician and have been here a very long time. I know everyone on the medical committees and I was Dean too.
>
> *DGM (ex-doctor):* I was chair of the medical advisory committee . . . Of course that background happened to be just right . . . and when the doctors here bring out the emotive element, they realize they are talking to an equal, someone who knows.

But most of the new general managers had no clinical training at all. Despite ministers' efforts to encourage the clinical trades to apply for the new managerial posts, the vast majority stayed put. Most RGMs, DGMs and UGMs were drawn instead from the administrators who had served the old consensus management teams. What could be done to supplement their skills? Take nursing as an example. For all the doubts about the adequacy of traditional nurse management, two-thirds of English districts none the less appointed a nurse advisor at district level. The justification was the need for detailed technical, cultural and political knowledge of nursing if the new strategy for clinical care was to be fully implemented:

> *DGM:* Nursing advice at the district level is all about the big picture, advising the district on the nursing implications of the strategic issues – manpower, capital plans, etc. . . . At the very minimum, a DGM needs a nurse and a consultant on the executive board just for self-protection!
>
> *DDQ:* There is a second type of advice that is also essential . . . which is the global,

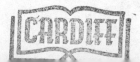

managerial view which is needed to make clinical nursing advice [from advisory committees or nurses lower in the organization] translatable for other people.

*CNA:* There's a political side to this job which needs my status. For example, it's theoretically possible that a UGM might be trying to pressure his DNS – then if she needs help, she can call me in; or, if I feel she's getting herself into a corner, then I'll step in . . . [And, on the other hand] nurses can't pull the wool over my eyes like they can over Jim's [a new UGM who had come into the NHS from industry].

*DCh:* We decided that in a district as complex and large as this, it was impossible to do without someone of Jill's [CNA] calibre. In fact, we haven't altered the structure Jill has created at all. She has a very good planning nurse; in fact all the support nurses are excellent. We haven't even discussed the question of not having DNSs. It's just not worth considering. People who talk of abolishing them must be mad. There's no problem there in this district.

*CNA:* I actually see the right skill mix and the right quality of care as being the professional advisor's role – whether they do it or whether they get someone else to do it . . . The central task is creating an environment for nursing, a sort of ambience for nursing which is seen as quality.

*CNA:* It's difficult to define [nursing advice] as I do it all the time and it takes place at so many different levels [but it's] expertise, safety, quality, planning and balancing all the things that have got to go on – for example, nurse education versus service constraints – and not just offering advice but practical solutions to problems that arise.

Even general managers with nursing qualifications could still feel a need for additional advice:

*DGM:* I talk to the DNSs in the units as they're involved in unit management, but I don't talk to them about staffing – that's Brian's [CNA] job . . . I'm not a general nurse by training, so professional nursing input to me on say, acute nursing, is a very important thing.

Creating a new professional advisory role was only part of the new approach to clinical care. A further strategy was to create an entirely novel district post, a director of quality. Such jobs were widespread in the new service. They were typically staffed by someone from the clinical trades, sometimes by the district medical officer, in one or two instances by an outsider such as an academic researcher but most often by a senior nurse. Thus, most quality directorships were held as 'hybrid' roles in tandem with the post of DMO or chief nurse advisor. And, here, as elsewhere, managers could appoint whoever they felt was most suitable for the job and give them whatever remit they felt was appropriate. Some quality directors stretched right across the traditional boundaries:

*DGM:* When nurses complain about quality, the thing is to see that we can get advice on this from the other quality experts in the district [the DMO was DDQ].

Some idea of the possibilities inherent in this new approach can be gained by considering the work of the quality directorate in a particularly innovative district. In this health authority, a sharp distinction was drawn between two sorts of clinical advice; that which the professions controlled and that which management controlled. A new professional nursing advisor had been appointed at unit level, a talented woman who headed a powerful and restructured advisory committee. But, in the new management structure, advice from the profession was sharply distinguished from advice about the profession. For the district general manager also had a separate quality director (an ex-DNO from another district) who reported solely to him:

> *DGM:* The person I look most to now for the best advice on district policy is Kate [district director of quality] . . . It isn't just the interpersonal skills you mentioned, it's the operational knowledge of the service. She understands the system . . . She advises *me*, not the authority. The difference this makes is, first that there's a clear division between advice to management and professional advice to the authority and second, that she's my girl – she's not facing split loyalties.
>
> *INT:* But it's expensive. Why create such a post?
>
> *DGM:* I have a treasurer to tell me about money and a personnel director to tell me about personnel. I also want someone to tell me about the quality of the product . . . I want Kate to tell me where nurse staffing levels are unsafe, where there's good nursing practice that can be used elsewhere – and where there are nursing practices that I should be worried about.
>
> *INT:* But how can she handle doctors?
>
> *DGM:* I expect her to come to me and say, just for example, 'Do you realize this operation is useless!' Then gently but firmly we'll tiptoe into the area. I'll get Kate to dig up the literature and then she'll say to the surgeons, or perhaps the MAC, 'This is terribly interesting – and of course, if we could save a million you could have the other consultant you want and some more beds. What a pity!'
>
> *INT:* And what if they object?
>
> *DGM:* I'll refer it to the quality panel. [The panel consisted of members of the health authority. The quality director was its secretary.] The members don't require too much to light the touch paper. They'll say, 'We pay the bill!'

## Conclusion: a permanent revolution

This and the previous chapter have reviewed the many dimensions of Griffiths. It was, as we have seen, a radically new approach to the organization of health care. At its heart lay a challenge to the syndicalist notion that the clinical trades knew best. That model was to be replaced by a very different order in which the new general managers took responsibility for that which had previously been lacking; a responsibility for the whole. This was, of course, a most ambitious programme, but that this was so was clearly recognized. For all the managerial enthusiasm for the bold new order, most general managers repeatedly stated that there would be many discrepancies between the dream and the reality and that its full implementation would take a very long time indeed. A total change in the outlook, training and vision of staff was required. New formal structures were only the start:

> *DGM:* My authority has welcomed Griffiths very enthusiastically. But . . . we see it as a marathon race rather than a sprint race.

*RNO:* What's not understood is that it's a totally different culture. It'll take ten to fifteen years . . . People still say to me that *committees* are the solution! I say, who cares how it's done; it's the performance that counts. We still haven't got it across yet. [Original emphasis]

Moreover, so it was stressed, not only was a completely new type of occupational culture involved, but many of the new techniques were only in their infancy:

*NHSBM (addressing an audience of finance directors and doctors):* We have a very distinguished team here today from Johns Hopkins. [An American hospital which was a leader in the development of new techniques for costing clinical care] . . . The prime aim of getting them here is to listen to what they've managed to achieve and [think about] what is applicable to us, as we struggle – and I think that's a fair word – through the various quagmires associated with management budgeting.

*DFD:* Quite clearly, nursing quality is a priority issue – but we've really only just started to look at quality in a concerted way. In the past, people have talked about quality without being able to prove it. A reasoned debate needs this.

In addition, not only were many of the ideas in their infancy but there was also – as we have repeatedly stressed – considerable district variation in the way they were applied. In the Griffiths vision, local managements were encouraged to experiment with very different solutions according to local need, capacity and preference. Take the examples of nursing advice cited earlier. English districts were free to decide on the precise location of the new nursing advisor. Most districts decided that a CNA was needed at district. But one-third of districts did not. They believed that advice should come from nearer the sharp end, down at unit. Attempts to argue otherwise were simply manifestations of the old tribal claims:

*INT:* What is the nursing role as regards professional advice?
*RM:* Bloody unintelligible! It's all they've got to hang on to! It's a load of cobblers in terms of corporate advice in DHAs and RHAs. If you want professional advice from nurses – say if you need to build a new hospital, which we really do – you can get it just for that particular job. To pay £25,000 a year for it is a disgrace. Professional advice is a load of hogwash! The only justification for them in management team positions has been the power of the profession. It's always been a spurious accident to have nurses at senior levels . . . The definition of the DNO role was so vague; the RNO role is even vaguer.

Such views were shared, though expressed slightly differently, by some nurses. Where the experience of district nurse management had been bad, not only the district general manager but even the senior unit nurses might be sceptical about the value of a continuing nursing presence at district. A nurse advisor based at district talked about the attitude of his colleagues to the new system:

*CNA/DNS:* Really, we have never had a lot of support staff at district anyway . . . Because of that, he [DGM] doesn't believe that having any more would help . . . To be honest with you, nursing here has had a very low profile for a long time. I did argue with my [nursing] colleagues when the structures first came out . . . that there needed to be nurses in [district] manpower planning . . . they disagreed with me. I was outvoted because they had experienced such poor service from nurses who pretended to be personnel officers . . . [that they] thought they would [now] benefit from a generic person.

Not only was the organizational style new, experimental and locally varied, but it had also to be recognized that the problems themselves never stood still; that no organizational solution could ever be complete. A central part of the new philosophy – so the prophets of Griffiths repeatedly argued – was an assertion that change was a constant and that staff had to be trained to cope with the consequences. Griffiths itself was only a beginning and there would be no end:

*BM:* Change – the key to my particular way of thinking about change is that it's my responsibility to get it into the culture of the organization. No one likes change all the time. We like to get into particular ways of doing things. We feel more comfortable that way . . . You have to move down the organization so that everyone in it has a responsibility for change. Whenever I meet people at different levels in my organization, I always put change on the agenda – under several different headings. I ask how they're changing the business to make it better and more profitable.

*DFD:* Jim [DGM] has spent a year of his time talking to nurses, doctors, paramedics – and to my staff as well – to really bring them along with the new changes. Even if he didn't always know what the changes were going to be at that time. Moreover, when the answers do appear, they won't be for ever. Things change all the time and the new structures might only be for a couple of years – because the problems change.

Griffiths, therefore, might 'form the framework of what we're trying to do', as one member of the NHS management board put it, but it was simply a framework, merely a starting point from which fresh structures and approaches might evolve:

*DGM:* My general feeling is that general management is too good to go. But the structures we've got now will evolve. I don't know where they'll go. It depends on the organization, on staff development and on the environment.

*DDQ:* My job wouldn't transfer . . . Where I'm really influential is in talking to Frank [DGM] . . . I had a real down recently. [I was thinking that] Frank will move on. There's no doubt about that. He could become an RGM in a couple of years' time. He trusts me and we work really well together, we counteract elements in each other. He's hard nosed, I'm too soft but that is a creative conflict and we have respect for each other.

*DFD:* I think Charles had had unhappy experiences of DNOs. I can't say I would have wanted one really. If we don't want one, what do we want? In a sense the solution evolved.

*DGM (in a district where nursing advice was now given part-time by a DNS at unit level):* Three years is a mere twinkling of an eye in the history of the health services and nursing needs that time to adjust to the new type of advice that's needed. They need time to become management oriented rather than just looking inwards to their peer group . . . In a year or so's time . . . we might go back to having a full-time CNA.

*CNA:* One of the things that I had hoped to achieve but don't think I will ever achieve is that we wouldn't have to have a hassle every time this post became vacant. But I think in fact that there will be a hassle each time it becomes vacant because it's the nature of the . . . structure below which is going to determine what you need at this level . . . We've got all new DNSs in post and in two or three years' time they could cope quite admirably. This post will always be subject to scrutiny.

Griffiths, then, was not simply a revolution; a mighty upheaval to be followed, when the dust had settled and the bodies been buried, by a new status quo. It offered instead a very different scenario; not Lenin but Trotsky – the possibility, indeed the necessity, of permanent revolution. This was doubly ambitious: both a mission into unknown territory and, simultaneously, an attempt to devise organizational methods so flexible and yet so robust that they could cope with any unforeseen eventuality. The future, so it was hoped, was built into the structure.

# PART 4   A LOOK AT DISTRICT

# History, locality, capital stock

Though a national service, the NHS was, just as crucially, locally run. Most doctors, managers and nurses worked not in Whitehall but in villages, towns and cities; in clinics, hospitals and headquarters which each possessed their own local history, their own social and economic circumstances. Thus, despite some fundamental uniformities, the service also varied in the most extraordinary number of ways. Such variation had a fundamental influence on the Griffiths reforms. The disparity between the way districts used nursing advice was not peculiar; everywhere one looked there was diversity. Writing for a trade paper, one district chairman noted:

> The five hundred or so [performance] indicators that have been circulated to each DHA show, it seems, 191 local health services rather than a National Health Service which operates in 191 districts.[1]

Thus, while Griffiths may have been a revolution, it was also the product of evolution, superimposed upon and massively shaped by the legacy of the local past. That legacy took very different forms in different places. Such variation is the main theme of the fourth part of this book. In this and the following two chapters we examine the great variety of local circumstance; a fact so fundamental that any reorganization had necessarily to be interpreted according to the practical demands of the immediate context. General management was moulded and transformed by the thousand and one details of local history, geography, demography, custom and industry. Despite this, the new administration offered, so its adherents claimed, a superior mode of coping with local variation; a method that both encouraged experiment and adaptation while simultaneously monitoring their actual success.

Yet, of course, although much of Griffiths turned on micro-management, on devolution, flexibility and responsiveness to local need, the NHS was still, as it had been from its inception, organized and administered from Whitehall. Whatever the local diversity, each unit, district or region still had to obey a host of regulations imposed from above. There were national rules about the composition of health authorities; the place of DMOs and CNAs; the appointment of chairmen, RGMs, DGMs and UGMs; the review of performance and the control of capital spending. When managers' thoughts turned to the frontline, they were faced by nationally organized occupations paid according to nationally determined scales, each presenting problems which were national rather than local in origin. Medical syndicalism, nursing hierarchy and general management were all national forms. This tension between national and local demands will form a key theme in the final part of the book. In this part, however, we focus on the local scene.

To do this, we examine the service from the viewpoint of district. In any large organization, the problems of size, complexity and distance force the construction of distinct tiers or layers of management between those in charge of the whole organization and those in the frontline. Given the size of the NHS, it too needed several layers of management and over the years a variety of tiers were created – regions in 1948, areas and districts in 1974, units in 1982 (the same year as the area tier was abolished). Districts, as we have seen, came in the middle of the NHS, halfway between the ward and the Secretary of State.

Based on a distinct geographical location and a defined local population, a district grouped together different types of medical and nursing facility. The task of each district's managers was to plan a coherent local health service with the particular staff and institutions which they had at their disposal. The typical district had at its core an acute hospital (a DGH) and, surrounding this, various forms of chronic, long-term and community-based care – a geriatric, psychiatric or a mental handicap hospital, health visitors, district nurses, well-baby clinics and so forth. All this looks neat enough. But, in reality, there was no such thing as a typical district. Psychiatric and mental handicap hospitals were often shared by more than one district. Some districts had more than one acute hospital. Districts which contained medical schools (teaching districts as they were known) had a variety of extra services. Rural districts sometimes had several tiny, local hospitals run by GPs, known as cottage hospitals.

Like every human institution, districts looked different from different standpoints. The phrase, district health authority therefore had several different meanings in NHS jargon. From an administrative point of view, a district was simply a management tier. But in another, more concrete sense, a district referred to the population and location served by a particular district health authority and to the hospitals and services that were used to this end. In this chapter, we consider both meanings – the abstract, administrative view as well as the particular features of different districts' size, history, wealth, industry, population, aspirations and capital stock.

District health authority also had a further meaning; it referred not to the population or the services, but to the chairman and to members of a special committee. That committee, the health authority, met once a month, reviewing the work of a district and setting its future policy. Its membership consisted, in key part, of local notables drawn from different sections of the community who served the same function as external directors in a private sector company. Thus, while the service may have been controlled by national politicians, it was also designed to respond to local interests and liaise with other local services.

Chapter 8 considers the influence of the wider community upon the service –
the influence of the local members, of the local press, of the local voluntary
groups, of the local politicians, of the local council and of the local authority
services which each council ran. All of these played a vital though varied part in
the shaping of local NHS management.

District also and lastly referred not just to the general administrative tier or to
the members of the health authority, but to the particular local bureaucracy – to
the managers of an individual district and the buildings in which they worked.
We start Chapter 9 by moving inside district headquarters, inside the converted
wards and Victorian houses, to examine the nature and quality of the new
district management; a quality that often varied just as much as that of the old
clinical management and which could present just as many problems.

We close Chapter 9 by examining just how the new order of Griffiths was
applied in particular local conditions. We sketch, very briefly, some of the
powerful ways in which local circumstances shaped the creation of very different sorts of management structure. But, if that is our conclusion, we must
begin with the circumstances. We turn, first, to consider districts' history,
location and capital stock.

## District origins

In the NHS management structure, each tier was subject to the tier above. The
first and most crucial power held by the tiers above district was geographic.
New districts could be called into life while others were divided or swallowed
up by their neighbours. At the same time, although every district was distinct,
each might sometimes have an important impact on its neighbours. Thus, what
looked neat on a national chart of the service, might look rather different from a
local point of view:

RGM: We built that new hospital – and got it under way – and X region took it off
us. All we got in return was Y district and a lot of problems.

CNA: The big problem region has had is Z district – creating a whole new district
with money that had to be transferred from all the other districts. It's created
horrendous financial problems for everyone. They've tried to play fair, but there
have still been very big disputes.

DGM: One thing that makes me wonder about how long we will survive as a
district is the fact that our DGH is actually located in a quite separate district . . .
This is why local people were so opposed to our closure of The Infirmary . . . We
were in fact linked to A district at one stage. We were split apart a few years ago.
You could actually split this district up and give bits to A, B, and C districts.

DNS: In London, we can plan for *our* needs, but then the surrounding hospitals close
their doors to admissions and we get all *their* emergencies flooding in. [Original
emphasis]

CNA: Gordon [DGM] is always knocking X district because they have all the
glamour [as a teaching district] and we do all the work. We don't have waiting lists –

except for ENT. And we are actually doing the work of the medical school because we have a lot of medical students here. There's lots of tension with region over this. Gordon is always fighting region over this.

Not only did each district, therefore, have a rather different relation with its fellows and masters, but some felt they should have no master at all. Up until 1974, teaching hospitals had been quite outside the geographic structure of command and were administered en bloc as a separate authority. Freed from such local ties, they had possessed even more independence; something their managers still fondly recalled:

> *DCh:* This district is a bit of a law unto itself. [Before 1974] it never regarded itself as part of the NHS! . . . Teaching hospital districts shouldn't be in regions. They should get funds direct from the Department. So one does feel frustrated.

> *CNA:* History is very important. Most of this district wasn't controlled by region. So there are grudges that go back a number of years. The relationship after 1974 was very awkward. We thought we'd lost something.

Geographical boundaries were not the only way in which districts might be treated differently by the tiers above. On some matters, Whitehall left regions to decide what was best for the tiers below. Some regions ruled with a very firm hand; others left districts to themselves. Take nursing, for example:

> *CNA:* This region has been one of the worst of all regions in the grading of its DNEs and educational staff . . . When it was nationally decided to bring the educational side into line with the management side, each region was left free how to interpret this. This region has been by far the meanest – living up to its reputation as one of the worst to nurses.

> *RNO:* I came here from X region where there were huge differences in the ranking of region, area and district. But here I was more the leader of a team. If they didn't like it, they didn't do it. It was more democratic.

> *CNA:* The relationship with the RNO is obsolete, it's defunct – and let me tell you something, it always was. I have never been to a regional nursing officers' meeting with all the CNOs sitting around the table, where I have seen any sense come out of it . . . The problem was that there was no specific reason why anyone should have backed a corporate view. Each CNO was a member of a separate district management team; there was no line management . . . I personally believe that the regional hand should have been strengthened. There was this mythical thing called advice, but no power went along with it. Don't let's perpetrate roles for the sake of it. If you look at the district personnel officer, well there was a very strong link between the DPOs and the RPO; they worked corporately. And it was the same with the treasurers. They were lateral thinkers while the small-minded nurses hid behind 'You can't tell me what to do!'

Districts, then, differed radically in their geographical and administrative history, in their sense of physical security, in their neighbours and superiors. Moreover, as we shall now see, each contained an enormously varied hotchpotch of buildings, services, staff and clientele, all of which – in their turn

– possessed their own distinct histories, memories, resources and plans. No district was the same as any other.

## A little, local difference

From a local perspective, Griffiths was merely an episode in the decades that it might take to build up a particular service, construct a new hospital or close another. General management might hasten or prolong the building of the new DGH, or the repair of the old one, but it was a force that only partially impinged on other developments, each with their own distinctive rhythms and timescales:

> *ML:* The objectives of a district don't change just because we've introduced general management. They stay the same. We said in introducing general management that what general management can do is aid and help the fulfilment of a district's objectives. General management is not an end in itself. General management is a new means to the old ends.

Those ends could differ very considerably indeed. Consider two extreme cases of the variation that could exist between districts:

> *DGM:* Take a look at this map. The district has got four and a half million sheep, it's a hundred miles long and fifty miles wide and it's got very little unemployment, except for this one valley here. Our main problem in this district is communication!

> *CNA:* This district has the problem of a very large ethnic population a lot of whom are very poor, there are a lot of single-parent families and a high rate of unemployment. We've also got twelve gypsy campsites within the district . . . 60 per cent of our nursing staff are black.

Thus, massive variations in location, ethnicity, size and the local economy all shaped the particular mix of problems that was faced by any individual district. In this complex stew of social and economic variables, one particular ingredient gave a flavour to all the rest. The capital stock – the physical plant – was the single greatest influence on the life of each district. Some districts had ancient, often widely scattered premises, others had a vast and brand new DGH. Some possessed huge, Victorian, psychiatric and mental handicap hospitals, often severely decayed, serving many different districts; others had a brand new laundry, or modern central cooking and stores facilities which offered services beyond the district. Some were the proud possessors of prestigious and highly expensive teaching hospitals, a few still had numerous, small community hospitals. Thus, the particular buildings and services that a district possessed shaped its management focus with a power that no other factor came near to approaching. Here, necessarily, was the place where management ended up most of the time.

## The acute sector

In all this variation, there was still one kind of uniformity. Most districts were dominated by their acute services. DGHs had all the thrill of curative medicine and the glamour – and expense – of high technology. Psychiatric, mental handicap and community services had far less prestige and attracted far less investment. Whatever the ideal preferences of managers or politicians, the acute sector was where most money ended up being spent:

> *CNA:* The UGMs don't like The Royal [DGH]. They think it's robbing Peter to pay Paul.

> *DNS/Asst UGM:* She [DGM] thinks of us [DGH] as the Palace on the Hill! She thinks that we've got more than we need.

> *CNA:* Most of our consultant appointments are linked to X [teaching hospital] . . . and there is great impetus to get academic units here if the university will transfer them. By contrast, the community sector has no teaching function, no GP training scheme and is medically very weak. So there's no championing of this sector at all. All the talk about switching the emphasis to the community has been so much talk.

> *Community UGM:* These [cuts] mean that the district is The Royal [DGH]; that there's nothing else in the district . . . It's actually very difficult in the present climate to put resources into services that are not capital led – so we're cutting health visitors and district nurses . . . I think we ought to take out a few consultants. Is the maintenance of acute services really sacrosanct when we've got some of the shortest waiting lists in the country, a growing population and falling community services?

But even if the community sector always lost out, there was still some variation in the extent and manner of its domination by other, more capital-intensive parts of the service. The acute sector normally had first priority within a district. But there could be exceptions. Even within the acute sector there were major variations in the size and shape of the priorities that it imposed. We have already seen the extreme contrasts that could occur between one district based in a deprived, inner urban area and another situated in a remote and rural part of the country. In the first, capital was concentrated in a large new DGH. In the second, it was dispersed across a dozen, small community hospitals. Each, therefore, involved very different sorts of management problems.

Such extremes were obviously rare. The power of the capital base to shape each district in a unique fashion is perhaps best shown by comparing far more similar districts. Both of the districts described below were primarily urban; both were non-teaching districts; both had a very large acute sector with ancient capital stock which absorbed most of the efforts of the new general management. Yet despite these important similarities, the particular details of capital construction, condition and location imposed their own distinct focus. The first district had a new DGH opened in the 1970s and was now trying to reconstruct the other, much older acute hospital. In the second, the rationalization of the old Victorian plant was at a much earlier phase:

> *DGM:* This time last year there was a lot of financial pressure on the district. We got caught on three things . . . We'd been very successful in reducing costs . . . so successful that we started the development programme six months early and this had serious knock on effects in the next financial year . . . Our cash runs in April were

twice the normal size . . . [Another] thing was the move to the [new] central stores which meant a huge first phase of requisitioning. Eventually, of course, reordering went way down, but in the very short run it has had the very reverse effect to what was intended. What should have been costs of £3 to £3.5 million in the first two months were in fact around £6 to £7 million . . . Another thing, the roof of The Southern [the 1970s' DGH] has been leaking . . . As a result, we've had to close theatres and beds and this has had a dramatic effect on waiting lists . . . We're going to go through exactly the same thing this year. We're going to have to close the theatres and the X-ray department for six weeks while we repair the other floors.

*CNA:* Acute services were spread over three sites here, separated by two main roads – at present we can't get patients from one site to another without road transport, they're very fast roads – and a fourth site a mile down the main road. This caused colossal logistical problems. It was a major contribution to our expenses . . . That process began in 83. The process of change has been very dramatic over the last couple of years. Our expenditure had to be reduced by something like £5 million. It was huge and it all had to be found out of the acute unit. So in the district strategic plan we arrived at the idea of relocating all the acute services, so as to reduce the number of buildings and sites in use. By 1994 we shall be on two sites only, linked to each other by a bridge. This will enable us to release a good deal of running costs and redevelop the other sites.

There were other, equally important differences within the acute sector. Huge institutions, such as hospitals, made enormous demands upon the local labour market; indeed, they were often the largest local employer. Yet that labour market could vary enormously between one part of the country and another. There was, therefore, yet a further major contrast between the two acute hospitals we have just mentioned. One, based in London, had increasing difficulties recruiting nursing staff. The other had few, if any problems. Such differences were fundamental to the service that was on offer:

*CNA:* In comparison with the inner London hospitals running at 20 and 25 per cent [nursing] vacancy factor, we're running at 15 per cent. So we are a damn sight better than Hammersmith and Paddington. But it is not good because 15 per cent is worse than last year when it was in single figures. The trend is rising.

*DNS/Asst UGM:* [When I was] at X [London teaching hospital] there was a very rapid turnover of ward sisters. The average stay was about three years. I came here and was amazed to see all these ward sisters coming up for retirement . . . At X there was always a continual struggle over staffing. Nights were held together by agency nurses but here there's no difficulty in recruiting. At one time, there was a bit of difficulty in getting relief nurses on nights, but that's changed with growing unemployment. There's not even a problem with geriatrics.

Moreover, where there was a shortage, nurses were not the only vital group in short supply. Consider this extract from a meeting of the main management group in another district where the labour market was tightening. The topic was the government's new policy of privatizing hospital cleaning services, something which had previously been done in house:

*DPD:* 'Bonus schemes' – the title is just a disguise. We're actually looking at the scope for further competitive tendering . . . We got away with it in the past because we said, 'Well it is a government directive'. But I don't think it will work so well with this. What kind of staff could we recruit on the basic rate? . . .

*DED:* Market forces are catching up with us. We can't recruit at the current rates of pay now. If we set the rate below that we'll fall apart . . .

*DPD:* My main worry is that it would be seen as industrial action paying off. Could we do as X district have done and leave the threat of competitive tendering there?

*DGM:* Would we actually attract any cleaners given Brian's [DED] emphasis upon current market forces? And it's very unattractive work. The place [mental hospital] is dirty and there are violent patients.

*DED:* It's a very close community.

*CNA:* That's right and that's why it works at the moment. Would it – if the current cleaning staff were got rid of and replaced by staff from all over the place?

*DGM:* Have we received any government pressure on this yet?

*DFD:* No.

*DGM:* I'd be inclined to keep mum about this one . . .

*DFD:* . . . But at some point we will have to demonstrate that we have tried to put things out to tender – though we can make the tendering documents so complex that people won't tender! There are ways round this.

*DGM:* Keep hanging on until the next election.

*DED:* We can say there's no need to change because we're decanting people from the hospital.

*DGM:* That's the line I'd go for.

Yet a further important difference between acute hospitals lay in the presence or absence of a medical school. As we saw in Chapter 2, the so-called teaching districts were a special case. From the viewpoint of general management, it was often a good deal easier to control both doctors and nurses in the absence of the imperious demands of a medical school. On the other hand, in some non-teaching districts, quality might suffer badly. Teaching hospitals could mean trouble with powerful clinicians, but they might also produce a service of which management could feel proud. Here was another source of major variation:

> *DGM:* In one respect, this district is better off than teaching districts in that not all our doctors are out to do wonderful things – I think in fact some of them are pretty mediocre.

> *CNA:* The medics here are pretty low quality. In fact, one of the Royal Colleges has just done a site visit and threatened to withdraw recognition from the trainees. This would be a disaster.

> *RNO:* About ten years ago, the standard of nursing was very heavily criticized by the doctors in X [a teaching district]. There was a medically inspired mandate for change – and even money for new nursing appointments. It only happened because it was a teaching district.

Even within the teaching sector there was important variation. In particular, the concentration of teaching hospitals in London meant that their interests dominated a good deal of the management of the four NHS regions into which the capital and the south-east of England were split; a dominance that caused considerable resentment amongst those on the outside:

> DGM: The crisis in London is really brought on by themselves. It's all caused by the teaching hospitals. The crisis in London is only a crisis if you assume that the teaching hospitals should be doing everything that they are doing.

Finally, though every district faced tight cash limits, there was fundamental variation in the capital spending which each was allowed. If every district was being squeezed, some were pressed far harder than others. Some districts, long mired in poverty, were now benefiting massively from RAWP – the scheme for redistributing funding from one part of the country to another – while other, much richer districts had lost out. Such variations in funding had fundamental consequences for the capital stock. Those districts that were gaining were expanding what they had. Those that were losing were cutting back:

> CNA: The capital programme here is vast because we're a major beneficiary of RAWP. This district was one of the poorest districts in the poorest region. Now the money is pouring in.

> DGM: We've had eight years of constant financial crisis here [due to RAWP] . . . really, I've become an officer for closures.

Thus, though clinical power and capital stock typically ensured the dominance of the acute sector, that dominance took a very different form in different districts. The exigencies of RAWP, of district size, of medical training and of the age, location and condition of the plant all led to major variation.

## Long-term care

The lesson of local variation is reinforced if we consider how, on occasion, the long-term institutional care sector might challenge the dominance of the acute service. Some districts had huge psychiatric and mental handicap hospitals which served many other districts besides the one they were in. In the 1960s there had been a series of major scandals in some of these hospitals – patients had died or suffered grievously as a result of their maltreatment by staff. As a result, a new national investigative body had been created and every such hospital was a potential worry for local management. Indeed, in one large, urban district with major problems in nursing recruitment, such a hospital at times threatened to swamp the district's other proceedings:

> DGM: When we had the Mental Health Commission Act report, they [region] did treat it as a matter of some serious concern, some priority, and one of my objectives is to persuade the RGM at our annual review meeting that we've actually now got the matter in hand.

> INT: It is extraordinary how we keep coming back to the care of the mentally handicapped . . . [Is it] . . . because it has been so long neglected . . . or is it because there is such a threat to mental handicap nursing?

> CNA: I don't think it's either of those. It's the fear of the members and the chairman

and the DGM that if anything is going to give us a bad press it's mental handicap. I think it is purely and simply that . . . The chairman does occasionally say, 'We must stop addressing the issues in mental handicap, we have an acute unit there which we are in danger of neglecting because every issue in mental handicap hits the press – and it's always a bad press'. I do think that in districts that do have a large institution like that, their acute units get shoved into the background.

Not every such hospital achieved this level of prominence. In one rural district, the concerns were of a very different order. None the less, such institutions remained a permanent background worry and past experience of similar places might still haunt managers:

*CNA:* I had a meeting here yesterday and the acting senior nurse from down there [MH hospital] said, 'Mrs Fox, we had three deaths in a week last week', and added, 'all natural causes'. I said, 'I'm glad to hear it!' . . . I remember Dr James from region going to the [MH] hospital – which really is, if there is such a thing, it is a sub-regional dump for the profoundly physically and mentally handicapped of all areas . . . and he said to me, 'How do you sleep at night with a place like that on your patch? It's so far away you can't see what's going on.' And I knew that I did [sleep well] and I had to think, 'Why do I?' and it is to do with the monitoring system. I had a place like that in X district – it wasn't for the mentally handicapped, it was for the elderly and I jolly well didn't sleep then. I mean I knew that was a bad place because the staff went off after their shift, they disappeared, they had no continuing relationship with their patients . . . [but] if you look at the turnover rates [of nursing staff] here [throughout this district] they are extraordinarily low, something like 3 per cent and most of those are retirement. Now that can be a bonus.

So major long-term institutions were another massive form of capital stock which had the power to shape a district; although that power was not wholly intrinsic but increased or diminished with other local factors. One such, as we have seen, was the ability to recruit a stable workforce. Yet another was the power of the staff. Just as teaching hospital doctors had more power than their brothers and sisters in the ordinary DGHs, so psychiatric and mental handicap nurses were far more solidly organized than their nursing colleagues elsewhere. Vast, isolated, under-resourced and neglected institutions staffed largely by men might sometimes, where local conditions were right, breed very powerful unions. Of course, compared to medical syndicalism, nursing trade unionism was often feeble. But in at least some institutions, they were a dominant force:

*DNS/Psychiatric UGM:* My main problem is how to get management in at all into this place!

*CNA:* There's been a very active branch of COHSE running to the press with stories . . . A lot of mischief making by trade union officials. The managers and the consultant haven't stood up to COHSE. The administrator is now the UGM and the one strong individual has given up the fight. COHSE have only been effective where there's been weak management and they've filled a vacuum – and in the late seventies this was undoubtedly the case. Management thought that by throwing money at it and listening to COHSE's endless grievances it would be OK. When the new management came in in 1981, conflict was inevitable.

*CNA:* COHSE have never been strong in mental handicap here and in mental illness the activists are very left wing and therefore have no sympathy for the membership. But nationally, there's a number of units I can think of where COHSE – well, it's very much like Murdoch and the print union – it's all come out in a number of inquiries. COHSE's strategy always tends to be no change at all. There's a whole lot of sons in the union – it's sometimes almost hereditary – entire families went into the job. [Our psychiatric hospital], however, has always had a philosophy of change. It goes back to the forties. So it's never been a problem here.

## District aspirations

Districts therefore had an extraordinarily varied capital stock. Some possessed a new DGH on a single site; others a multitude of community hospitals, an internationally famous medical school, a scatter of ancient decaying buildings, or a vast Victorian warehouse for the mentally or physically infirm – or various combinations of all of these. Districts also varied in size, industry, population, culture and wealth. Given such variation, the standards to which they aspired were extremely diverse. A few might aim to be the very best. Such districts could attract the best staff and engage in not just one but in many different experiments. Moreover, rich, powerful and prestigious districts like these could, if they so wished, take an independent line, speaking to the public, battling against region, nobbling ministers. Teaching districts, in particular, had enormous independent powers of influence:

*DFD:* This district is very high pressure and very low cost . . . We're big, exciting and efficient.

*CNA:* I genuinely believe we have some of the best DNSs and support staff in the country. So we can take risks where others can't.

*DFD:* I said [to him] that I thought we were the most cost-efficient district in the service and had the best consultants.

*INT:* (*smiles*)

*DFD:* It's true, we are the best.

*CNA:* The chairman's given up trying to influence the region. He goes national – straight there – to MPs and ministers direct.

*DGM:* Within this region, there's a couple of authorities that are almost renowned for members running to the press and trying to put pressure on the RHA in advance of RHA meetings, and saying that they've got to close wards, 'We've got to close this, we've got to close that'.

Such districts were rare. Slightly more common, perhaps – though still highly favoured – was another sort of district; situated in a small city in a rich part of the country and lacking the special problems that went with major conurbations. Such districts might lack the glamour of the big teaching hospital but in some respects had fewer problems, could still attract good staff and innovate in pleasant surroundings:

*CNA:* It's a very stimulating environment here. There's a great deal of support and there's a lot going on. And there's lots of interesting research and a whole lot of projects I can push on – the people are all so receptive.

*Acute DNS/Asst UGM:* It's a new hospital. People are very friendly. They welcome outsiders – some places don't. You do need an element from the outside, otherwise you get very incestuous and you don't know about the wider world. There's a very good standard of nursing care and a much more stable workforce than at X [London teaching hospital] . . . There are very good relations between the school and the service side here; much better. The school of nursing is extremely good. There are very high calibre students and we're involved in appointments. You also know much more of the district as a whole than you did at X. Because at X you never saw Cogwheel (medical advisory committee) minutes, you never knew the politics of the place. But here, it's much freer and more open. I don't know to this day whether X actually had any district plans! So it was a good decision to come here . . . The finance director's a sweetie. They're [district managers] all easy to talk to – that's another thing about this place, *even* the district people are friendly! [Original emphasis]

Most districts, of course, could not aspire to the big league, or afford independence. Their aim was simply to do better than they had done in the past, to be average:

*CNA:* One of the big problems is, do you raise standards when you can't really afford it? Whenever I try to talk to Sheila [DGM] about really good care, she just says to me, 'We're just an ordinary health authority trying to do an ordinary job for ordinary people. There are some health authorities that try to be centres of excellence, but we're not.'

*DGM:* Now we've actually decided, as a matter of some policy that – not necessarily that we grin and bear it – but that we certainly don't make a mountain out of a molehill . . . We could quite easily last year have closed wards. I mean we were £250,000 overspent and the fact that the pay awards were not funded and the fact that we'd not put enough in reserve, well we could have taken what I regard as quite easy options. But the hard options are to peg things back and to get an actual level of activity that the authority itself can contain.

Finally, far out along the spectrum were those other districts that were almost overwhelmed by long neglect and the poverty of their clientele; districts where the challenge was greatest but whose managers sometimes despaired:

*DGM:* I don't think the quality of service is very good in this district. It's not good in the medical, in the nursing or in the support departments. What's the cause? I've not been around as much as I'd like to have been, but I have got a feeling of low morale. There's a lack of commitment in some instances which I've not experienced before. The guts to get things going, well, it's just not there. It may be the calibre of the people who've been appointed – or it may just be the area. Though I'm not unhappy with the board appointments . . . [But] I worry, can we recruit the supporting network. I have the vision . . . the UGMs have the vision . . . and I can put the posts together – but can I fill them?

*DNS:* My first impression here was one of deprivation. It was that that attracted me. But my other impression was of how behind the times it is compared to the one I worked in before . . . Take the statistics. This sheet is called clinical returns. They indicate the number of people attending sessions. They don't say why people are there – which they do in other districts. So if they come for three things, they're just ticked once. And there's no computerization. In X district, we had hand-held computers, there's nothing here . . . When I suggested it people said, 'Nurses will never manage that!' I thought I was dreaming . . . So many of the staff were born here and will die here. They just don't want to change . . . When I came here I was stunned. Some people have been here fifteen years and never done a refresher course . . . What's needed is early retirement. We need new blood. There's no get up and go. Students just apply here because it's the place nearest them. There's no idea of acting by themselves or going out and exploring. I've taken some of my staff to meetings to show them new types of service that are being done elsewhere. They say, 'Well we're doing that here, we've been doing that all the time. We come out pretty well.' Absolute rubbish! We're not providing those services and never could . . . I've had to start from square one. I feel I'm going backwards . . . It's very heavy here politically . . . I've had a queue of people here complaining – partly about race and partly about religion . . . A lot of people come in and talk about colour quite openly . . . I didn't know before I came here that it was so important which island you came from . . . I've even had a Jewish health visitor complaining that Jewish families wanted Jewish home helps! We don't try and match religion though – it's hard enough trying to do it with race. I've had to establish my credibility as regards race. Actually, it happened quite by accident. I'd stuck up a whole lot of postcards and one of them was of a little black boy. It was taken as a sign of good faith. I'd stuck it up, along with a whole lot of others, because the room was so dreadful! . . . The district isn't so well off. On paper it's not so bad. You can get home helps any day of the week. But in practice the resources are poor . . . We don't even have a proper personnel department. There was no real guidance when I came here. I had to do everything myself . . . The politics feel tight right throughout the district. The social workers are always going on strike and when one section is out, the others won't take up the workload. We always support each other. They don't. So communication is very problematic with them. And they're not very experienced – they're straight out of college . . . X hospital is a disgrace. There's rubbish all over the place. It's an absolute disaster area . . . Quite honestly when I came here, I thought I'll do a year here and then I'll go. It's like an allotment that's never been turned over. And if you go away for a week, you return and it's a disaster all over again. It just reverts. It's like the tide – it goes out but it always comes back in again.

## Conclusion

Although the NHS was a national service, there were, then, huge local differences. The managers of a massively deprived inner-city district with very high levels of unemployment and a large immigrant population faced fundamentally different problems from those whose population was thinly scattered over a vast rural area. Both these, in their turn, were different from, say, a teaching district in an affluent part of the country or a district whose population was almost entirely suburban. And, even where districts' size and population were fairly similar, there were, as we have also seen, many other factors which could lead to important differences in some of the key tasks that faced local managers: the history of a district and its relationship to the regional tier above; its relative wealth and whether it stood to lose or benefit from RAWP; the position, age and condition of its hospitals; the presence or absence of vast long-term institutions; the state of the local labour market; the power of local trade unions. Such factors both shaped managers' tasks and dictated districts' aspirations. Grifiths might aim to provide a better service than had hitherto existed but, in any particular place, that vision of the future was necessarily tightly constrained by the myriad details of local culture, demography, economics, history and geography.

# Local politics

Now add even further complications. The thousand and one pressures which gave each district its unique shape included not just the inanimate factors of size, industry, the labour market and the capital stock but the more personal pressure of the local citizens and their various representatives. That pressure is the main subject of this chapter. Every district was politically moulded, in one way or another, by the local community. For a start, while each district served the health needs of its population, no health authority ran the necessary range of services to meet all those needs. Some vital services were provided by voluntary groups; others by the local council which, unlike the health authority was locally elected and thus (in key part at least) politically controlled by local, not national government. Moreover, the health services themselves, although nationally provided, retained an important element of local representation. Every district had its members: local men and women, whose job was to formulate the strategy that each authority took. Once again, all this led to considerable local diversity.

## Local news, local services

Since the health service was a huge local employer and every local citizen was potentially a patient, health service matters were a subject of keen local interest. The most immediate political pressure therefore came from the press. Ward closures, new hospitals, road accidents, fund-raising drives, suicides in the local psychiatric hospital and the miraculous survival of premature babies: the NHS, in one way or another, formed a major component of all local news. Just dealing with journalists could occupy a considerable portion of a general man-ager's time – though this varied according to the district's location. The mass media in large conurbations were far more numerous than those in rural areas:

> *INT:* So day to day decision making has gone down the line?
> *DGM (in inner urban district):* In the main . . . [Of] the things I keep up here [for myself], one is any major dealings with the press – so that actually from time to time causes a fair bit of activity and a fair bit of workload because you've got five or six newspapers and three radio stations telephoning you – or whatever.

Local pressure and voluntary groups, too, had to be managed with care. From 1974 onwards, such groups had been partially incorporated within the NHS via the creation of community health councils (CHCs). Their importance varied significantly from place to place and over time. Consider their role in two very different districts. The first quotation is an extract from the weekly meeting of a district management group. The item on the agenda was sheltered accommodation for the mentally handicapped:

SDMB: What about any CHC involvement [in these negotiations]?
DGM: I'd say no.
CNA: How would they react?
UGM: They're very sympathetic.
CNA: They've been very good to us over Y.
DGM: What do you think?
DCh: You can't have them on the negotiating team.
UGM: So I'll just tell them where we've got to.
DCh: Yes, you can tell them that – but we can't have them running things for us!

CNA: We had a very good CHC secretary. He gave us a really hard time! But it's not the force now that it was. The best thing about it then was that it was predictable. You knew you were in for a hiding! Now it's not predictable at all. Sometimes it's asleep for very long periods. Occasionally, it suddenly wakes up. For example, just recently, the CHC suddenly objected to some of our mental illness plans [to shut a large mental hospital] so it's gone to the Secretary of State. We'll have to wait and see if he dilutes them. These days everyone's a self-appointed expert on mental illness!

If the local press and local pressure groups kept a sharp, though varying focus on the activities of district, their significance was far outweighed by those local services on which the NHS depended but over which it had no control. Health care was merely a part of the local welfare state and in local government, the district health authority had a potential rival which was run according to its own distinct principles. Here too was a major source of diversity. Local government was shaped by the same powerful forces that moulded its counterparts in health – by local industry, geography, culture and demography. But unlike their brothers and sisters in health, the social services they ran were part of no central organization and were directly subject to local political control.

Despite this, there were still some things in common. Both sets of managers were unhappy with the conventional way services were split between them. Liaison was difficult between separate authorities. Long-term and community care fitted awkwardly with the acute health sector. Patients might be better served by new methods of integration. In 1974, for the very first time, a nationally ordered means of liaison was created. Joint consultative committees had been set up both to plan and to funnel money directly from the NHS into relevant social services. And to aid such formal symbiosis, the health service grew an extra tier – area – midway between district and region, which matched, as the others did not, the geographical boundaries of local government organization. Thus, in 1974 consensus planning became the order of the day not just within the NHS but between the NHS and the local authorities.

For all the high hopes that inspired these reforms, the methods were not a success. This administrative engineering had much the same faults, many argued, as consensus management within the health service. Power and performance were discreetly ignored. Despite the huge variation in organization, personnel, scientific traditions, methods of funding and political control, it was enough, or so it had been hoped, to state a common interest and create consultative machinery. Once the bureaucracy was in place, harmony would follow. In practice, there were manifold problems and huge variation in what was actually achieved. As a result, the area tier was abolished in 1982 and the attempt at geographical integration abandoned. Some progress was, however, still being made, though the way was hard. The great complexity of financial, institutional and staff collaboration in these matters is revealed in the following lengthy quotation taken from a meeting of a district's management board. The item on the agenda was the closure of the local mental handicap hospital:

UGM: We're moving towards closing The Heath in the summer. The numbers left now are too small to support a whole hospital. The idea has been to move the last people out into bungalows in X town. The environment there would be similar to that of the proposed accommodation in the city. That plan's still on but there are some problems . . . We need to shut The Heath now – some of the people left spend all day marching round the huge open spaces left there and making life very uncomfortable. [The UGM then explains her plan.]
DGM and DFD: [Engage in technical discussion of its financial implications.]
DGM: How much of this has been taken into account in the development costs?
UGM: It's not.
DGM: Well we haven't got it [the money] . . .
UGM: I think it can be done.
DGM: How?
DCh: Can you try and go through it again . . .
UGM: If we get on fast with it now, the county council should be able to fund the difference from social security.
DGM: Our total development money for next year is just £118,000. If we spend the £100,000 you want, it means another year when we're spending almost all our development money on mental handicap.
UGM: But what I'm saying is that we can't close The Heath unless we spend more money.
CNA: You're saying we either spend £100,000 now [on closing it and opening new accommodation] or we spend £12,500 a week on The Heath, which is £600,000 a year?
UGM: Paying for The Heath is a completely mad cost.
CNA: It must be more logical to spend £100,000 that we haven't got than £600,000 that we haven't got.
DCh: Thank you for putting it so concisely! . . . In cash terms what's the benefit that we would get from the county council?
UGM: The more we hand over, the more they can plough in. We'd pass over the revenue on funding for 23 staff [for the bungalows]. We'd staff those 23 and they'd top up on staff to the Wessex ratio of 40.
DCh: That seems marvellously advantageous.

*DEO:* It must be right, but the cost consequences of providing temporary accommodation could be enormous.

*DCh:* Surely not . . .

*UGM:* I don't know if you've been there [The Heath] recently but . . .

*DCh:* Yes, it's terrible . . .

*CNA:* We'll get huge advantages from it – a superb service. I think we should go for it.

*DCh:* Yes, go for it hard . . . We need to get a management team working now to provide continuity. Who should be on it? . . .

*UGM:* Do you want anyone from social services?

*DCh:* What's your advice?

*UGM:* Well! Ummm!! I've got a summary here of last week's meeting in which they expressed all their anxieties. They're worried that if things go wrong, will social services be held responsible. They want them registered as nursing homes!

*DCh:* Does dual registration apply?

*CNA:* No. It causes more conflicts because there are different sets of rules.

*UGM:* It's also more expensive.

*DEO:* These are just large hostels. They ought to be more consistent on logic.

*UGM:* But it's better to have them alongside us rather than glaring at us . . .

*UGM:* [Suggests a member from social services.]

*DCh:* Do you know the chairman of the council?

*UGM:* No.

*DCh:* Well I do, quite well.

*DGM:* He's as wet as that man in *Yes, Minister* about choosing bishops that was on the other night!

*DCh:* I think I'll try and square him.

*DPD:* Should we raise this at the joint chief officers' meeting on Wednesday? . . .

*CNA:* No. They'll be like rabbits in a car headlight with this one. They'll be terrified of the implications. It'll just give them warning . . .

*DFD:* I think it's sensible only to bring it to the authority when it's virtually buttoned up . . .

*UGM:* What about the personnel side, Jean [CNA]? It has been mentioned but we're awaiting more details.

*CNA:* I think I'll talk to Brian [social services officer] about this. I suspect they'll be interested if they're paid on care assistant scales rather than on our salaries . . . That would sell it . . .

*UGM:* What I've got from this meeting is two things: first that I set up a committee with X council; second that I prepare a paper with a rough draft of the negotiations.

*DGM:* Yes, just so that a few members are knowledgeable before the public meeting . . . We do need a clear financial paper on this one, Keith [DFD] because so many figures have gone round the table in the last half hour . . . Jim [CHC] informed me on Friday that the treasurer's job was an art.

*DFD:* It's a miracle, not an art!

In this district, then, there was progress, despite many tensions. But there could also be fundamental problems which limited the advance that could be made. Some councils were preoccupied with their own affairs:

*CNA:* The local authority began in 1982 by not putting a single elected councillor on – they hadn't got any time for the health authority. It took several years before they realized that they could get resources out of the health service and into the social services. Now, however, we've got the chair of social services on, a very strong character.

Serious divergences in methods of organization might also hinder liaison. Where one devolved, another might be centralized. Difficulties could occur in either direction:

> CNA: The local authority has embarked on a programme of devolution of town hall responsibility. They've carved the borough into fifteen sub-units, built expensive new office blocks, recruited hundreds and hundreds more people and broken down all their services to this level. This exercise has had enormous consequences for us. The lines of communication are now extremely complex – even the people on the council don't know how to get hold of the right people. It'll settle down eventually though.

> CNA: We feel that the social services department have not cooperated very well with us because they run things centrally and we have devolved. So it makes them very difficult to deal with. Their continual refrain is, 'I will have to refer that to my Director'.

Problems could also arise in divergent levels of funding for similar or closely linked services. Activity by one service could create problems for another, for their interests might well overlap. The precise boundary between health visitors and social workers was, for example, sometimes unclear:

> CNA: We've now got our health visitor surveillance of the elderly – that's been running a year . . . it has generated a whole lot of aggro with social services because, of course, it has thrown up a whole lot of need. They were asking us not to make referrals and I said, 'Sorry, what you do with the referrals is your business, but having found a need, we have to tell you about it' . . . I would be delighted if someone did my need finding for me, but they've really been very aggressive about it . . . They say that it has generated an enormous amount of need that they can't meet . . . They have got problems and in a way this is why we needed to do it because I think the social services spend 5.5 per cent of the county council expenditure on things like home help services against an area average of 7 per cent and an upper one of, say, 12 per cent. I mean, it's not my fault if they haven't got their resource distribution right.

Not every local authority was thought to be mean. In others the reverse was true. And in a few, the lavishness with which they spent caused grave fears about incompetence, possibly even corruption, at least to some on the district side. Here, for example is an extract from a health authority meeting. The item under discussion was a joint scheme to create sheltered housing for the mentally handicapped. The building work was being undertaken by the local authority but some of the health authority members had serious worries about the propriety of the borough council's actions:

> DCh: The next item is the Oaktrees project. It's now been agreed that the

Borough's direct labour department will do the contract for £250,000. Would you like to comment, Mrs Jones?

*Mrs Jones (member):* All I have to say, is 'God speed'.

*DCh:* Mr Haughey, would you like to say anything?

*Mr Haughey (member):* Yes, I want to comment and I want my comment minuted. In the end, this is a very unsatisfactory deal. Indeed, I want to add that this is one of the most unsatisfactory deals that I have ever been associated with. I want to read from *our* [district's] quantity surveyor's report on the tender. He says that it has so many qualifications written into it that it is impossible to ascertain how much it will cost. There can be no guarantees of anything . . . I could spend the whole afternoon reading out the qualifications. Our surveyor says that it's only because it has been explicitly guaranteed by the borough that the district could proceed with this project. [Original emphasis]

*Mr Briton (member):* . . . I object to what Mr Haughey has said. I don't normally disagree with him, but I do in this case. The health service is getting a bargain out of this through the JCC.

*Mr Haughey (member):* I just thought members ought to know that we are party to a deal of which, though our part is clear, the other part is not.

*Mrs Wallace (member):* You're behind the times, Mr Haughey. The contract has been approved.

*Mr Rose (member):* What happens if the ratepayers challenge this deal? Could we end up losing the building?

*DCh:* No, even if the party in power changed, we would have to honour the contract.

## Health authority members

The health authority members – such as those in the previous quotation – were, in principle at least, the people who steered each district's policy. Their rule was based on traditions that went deep into Britain's past. Modern health authority members still carried distant echoes of the patrons of the eighteenth century voluntary hospitals and of the local worthies who had met in the parish vestry from Tudor times onwards and administered the poor law. There were, however, some fundamental differences. Though the local merchants and gentry were still present, the NHS had made room for other representatives of the local community. Local councillors were now guaranteed a few places on the authority. A local trade union representative had also been admitted. At the same time and in line with health service syndicalism, the clinical trades were also represented, both doctors and (from 1974) the nurses too.

Every month, the district accounts were presented to a health authority meeting and reports on district policy were routinely discussed. Members also undertook tours of inspection and sat on appointments committees. Thus, the officers (as local managers were traditionally called) faced a double task: both managing the service and persuading the members that they were conducting that function appropriately. Despite members' nominal control of policy, their power was usually weak. Real clout typically lay with the officers, with doctors and with central government. None the less, members still had a powerful nuisance value for many managers and some made systematic efforts to block various health service reforms that had come from DHSS.

As a result, significant modifications to the system were introduced in 1982, changes which tied in closely to the centralizing, managerial thrust of the Griffiths reorganization. Chairmen were now paid, though on a part-time basis. In line with the increased monitoring of performance by central government, the Secretary of State now took a far more active interest in the nomination of chairmen and members – except for those of the local council representatives which lay quite outside the ministerial remit. Thus, although important el-ements of the old system remained, the power of chairmen had been consider-ably increased and that of the ordinary member had been reduced. One chairman commented wryly on the constitutional changes that had occurred in health authorities and their membership since the NHS was founded:

DCh: The old division into district, area and regional authorities was to accommod-ate the Morrisonian position as opposed to that of Bevan and in its early years it was very much the most marvellous piece of eighteenth-century patronage! Mind, there's still a lot of councillors involved. However, this government has at least introduced a few more professionals [on to the authority].

As this comment suggests, there remained a strong feeling amongst the new managers that, despite recent change, the system worked poorly and fitted badly with the effective running of the service. What actually was members' role and what did they know about health care? Were most local members simply too ignorant to play any sensible role?

CNA: It's the whole local approach. It's small-minded, parochial and more con-cerned with the nitty gritty than managing a £50 million a year business. It's run like the corner shop.

DFD: Members aren't elected and there's a lack of identity. The members' role post-Griffiths is very confused. Local authority members are absolute disasters be-cause they have very preconceived ideas about the NHS – and a lot, being snobbish, don't have the intellectual capacity. They need more training – which is very old hat. Having said all that, as an officer in a health authority [compared to working for a local authority] you do have a much better ability to take decisions – and the members have a more strategic role. Whereas local authority councillors can't let go. They make decisions on the colour of the walls! From 48 to 74, I think health authorities were much more like this.

DGM: Some members . . . a small minority, believe that it [Project 2000 – the plan to upgrade nursing education] is a cost-cutting exercise and that they are reducing nursing manpower! . . . Even though I have been at pains to emphasize that the nursing profession has put up a solution, [that] this isn't actually a political influence. At the moment, an awful lot of things are given political connotations which actually have no bearing. So what we've done is defer discussion on it until the next meeting.

CNA: One thing about the health authority that I loathe is the politics of it . . . . it's so stupid. I find it incredible. You see, they are monitoring us and they don't know what they are looking at, they don't know what they are talking about. I have asked if I can go with the monitoring panel when they visit St Hilda's – because all they're listening to is the UGM who isn't going to show anything he doesn't want to show. I find it quite incredible . . . The Cumberlege Report [suggesting an extended role for nurses in general practice] . . . was discussed at the health authority meeting at the same time as [a district] document on primary care which was mostly for medical staff . . . We [the officers] couldn't agree because the nurses' viewpoint was going to be one way and the GPs didn't actually want the Cumberlege recommendations. So we pointed out to the members that there was this conflict due to professional issues here . . . and, of course, the nursing one got nodded through and the primary care one – they tore it to shreds . . . I don't think it's a lack of concern, it's a lack of comprehension . . . [But] whenever we have education sessions they don't come.

Just as many officers had doubts about the members, so members, too, might worry about the role they were supposed to fill and their lack of preparation. Here, for instance, is an extract from one health authority meeting:

*Mr Joseph (member):* I find it very odd that as a new member, there's not a set of documents to fill you in. I feel you can probably only be an effective member if you've been here at least a couple of years.
*Mr Wardle (member):* I'm also fairly new and I'm unclear about what we're supposed to do between meetings and what our relationship with officers is supposed to be. I'd like some information on how other district authorities manage with their members in, perhaps, a more advanced sort of way. And how can we get some channel of communication with region? They send us all these outrageous statements. How can we get back at them?
*Mr Haughey (member):* I found the King's Fund training very valuable.
*Mr Alexander (member):* I did too but I'd also like to see some sub-committees and more seminars . . .
*Dr Griffiths (consultant member):* I'd find it difficult to manage a whole day's meeting . . . though I would certainly recommend perhaps spending a couple of days at the region's very nice conference centre!
*Mrs Jones:* Some of us remember doing this a very long time ago, don't we! (*looking at chair*)

Members, too, then, had worries about their role and the adequacy of their training. Likewise, many of them shared the nagging doubts about the system's adequacy as a method of public representation; a doubt that was reinforced in some districts by the absence of the public themselves at those meetings to which they were invited. Consider another extract from a health authority meeting:

*DCh:* This [proposed] meeting of the JCC is to be open to the public.
*Mr Wardle (member):* That's fine – but how can it be made more open to the public? We need to advertise it.
*DCh:* My own experience of local government is that the general public are never interested except, when it's a matter of very special concern, when you're closing something – they never turn up for anything new – or when it happens to be raining. This, unfortunately, is democracy as I have known it.
*DGM:* We do advertise in all the local papers.

*Mr Haughey (member):* We should move the meeting to my pub – we discuss everything there!

However, although there was, indeed, widespread concern about both the ignorance of the members and the apathy of the public, there was none the less very considerable variation between health authorities. Some were more active than others; some were more politicized; some made far greater efforts to involve the wider public. Since localities themselves differed so dramatically, the way in which that local interest was expressed could take extraordinarily divergent forms. At one extreme, for example, was a rural authority whose key members had sat there for many years, exerting great power over the life of the district. Only now, with a new set of managers and the retirement and resignation of the old members, were things beginning to change:

*DGM:* We're shortly going to lose some of the difficult members, thank God! And we've also got a dynamic new chairman . . . Before I came, the officers were just not prepared to take on the health authority . . . The deputy chairman has also just resigned. He couldn't take all the changes. He was totally opposed to the concept of community care. He just wanted all the old people shut away in hospital . . . They hadn't spent a penny on HQ since we came here sixteen years ago . . . Though there were three units in the past, in fact the members had had a very centralizing policy and had refused to devolve.

At quite another extreme were those authorities with a strong left-wing membership, as these quotations from two inner-city districts make clear:

*Asst UGM/DNS:* The health authority in this district impinges on the work much more than most – perhaps because it's a left-wing district . . . you have to be politically aware. It's not at the front, but it's definitely always at the back of my mind! For example, I was talking to a friend of mine. In her district, the health authority meeting starts at 10 am on a weekday and no members of the public ever go. Ours is at 5 pm and we always get lots of members of the public. If I made six auxiliaries redundant tomorrow, I'd have the health authority down on me like a ton of bricks!

*DCh:* The local council has got, in my terminology, a lot of loony lefties. In public, relations with them are deplorable – though in private they're not too bad! I take the flak and let the DGM get on with it behind the scenes. On the authority, the four council representatives and the trade union representative always vote together. In fact two of them look at the others to see how to vote because they can't follow the arguments! They always oppose value for money initiatives, rationalization, economy. They interpret it as sackings. I'm very much a VFM person. I'm not trying to save money – but I want to spend it on providing services, not just on providing employment.

Despite their power to vote on district policy, members' power was in some respects quite heavily restricted. They had to work within ministry guidelines and the initiative lay typically with the chairman, with the general manager, with doctors and officers, but not themselves. None the less, as the example of the rural district suggests, in some places members had been able to exert considerable influence. Moreover, in all districts, members could still exert an important influence in certain key areas such as appointments and hospital closures:

> *CNA:* The DNS post in the new unit was a real cock-up! On the appointments committee, there were two of the far left councillors . . . The problem was that Bill [the internal candidate] had told both of them in the past to piss off!
>
> *INT:* What are the major tasks for you at the moment?
>
> *DGM:* Well, we've got the medical staff absolutely committed to a one-site hospital and the health authority absolutely committed to a two-site hospital. [The acute services were currently on two sites.]

Thus, whatever their weaknesses, the members could not be wholly ignored. DGMs and chairs had to spend a good deal of time selling their policies. Techniques varied. Members rarely opposed most aspects of a district's strategy, but a few issues were highly sensitive and could require special care:

> *DCh:* [Apart from] the loony lefties . . . there are one or two overt Tories . . . I'm a Tory . . . and then there's a big middle ground of professionals . . . I've never had a party meeting beforehand – although occasionally I do phone people. But the council people [Labour] are mandated to take particular views. However, we have got competitive tendering through. The members voted it down, the Department said we would have to [do it]. So I blackmailed two of the members by saying region would cut our budget by what we ought to have saved – that nearly got the vote – and then I waited until two other members were on holiday and then called a meeting. Such is the way of government!

Members, then, could sometimes be manipulated; but not all relationships with members were so strained. In some authorities, as we have seen, the DGM and the chairman, or one of the two, made systematic efforts to involve members in decision making through a sub-committee structure, although not everyone approved:

> *CNA:* I didn't like the chairman at first, but now having seen X district [where the CNA is the nursing member on the authority], I really appreciate her. In X everything is decided in sub-committees. The authority is merely a rubber stamp. And unlike here, there is no place on the agenda for members' questions.

Sub-committees, however, could be used for serious democratic ends. A DGM or chair, although still believing in the importance of the members, might still set out to train and guide them in a highly systematic fashion. Once educated and steered in the right direction, a members' panel could ask awkward but useful questions, seemingly – and sometimes actually – of their own volition:

> *DGM:* Let me qualify the arrogance of my next statement by some comments from someone who was here and who is now a UGM in the North. She went there and was appalled by the level of the members' comments. She said, 'We need you here to take the members on for six months'. Because I've done that since I've been here . . . I brought the panel system [sub-committees] here from Y Area [area was the old

management tier between region and district created in 1974 and abolished in 1982]. When I arrived in Y, the only time the officers met the members was at the health authority meeting. It was regarded as a good day out by the DMT reps [the officers from the old district management teams]. We met in the afternoon and the name of the game was to have as much fun as they could at the expense of the area officers. The briefing for the chair took place only that morning! There was no agreed policy or anything. After the first few meetings, I changed all that. All the papers went through prior to the meeting. And I introduced a panel system at which only the area officers were present – so the DMT was excluded. There were two advantages. It gets more business done – because the members trust each other whereas they might not trust officers. The second thing is, if members present it, it tends to go through. The members thought it was wonderful when we introduced it here. No panel has executive authority so the members don't feel excluded. Our new DMO said there was a huge difference from his previous district where the officers did all the talking and the name of the game was to catch the officers out.

*DDQ:* I've been very pleased with the way I've managed to get the health authority's quality panel to look at the PIs [performance indicators] for each medical speciality . . . Of course, it's a very slow process as the panel only meets once every two months. But there are some good members, some of the sharper ones are very, very good – they latch on to the salient features right away.

Not every authority was so malleable. Some districts were faced with a hostile local authority armed with a new kind of political programme. The Labour Party had created the NHS and in doing so, had destroyed the extensive municipal health services. But, forty years on, a new mood had arisen within its ranks. In many Labour-controlled local authorities, the new political agenda aimed to abolish central control and restore local political power, putting health and social services on the same footing and under the same boss. Officers in such districts could thus face consistent opposition both from the local authority and from the council members on the health authority. Yet, even in such circumstances, there were important local variations. In one district, faced with determined opposition from the council, the general manager contemplated revenge:

*DGM:* Relations with the local authority are no better. Collaboration is no better at all. They claim to be interested in collaboration but in fact they want to take over the health service. The first major collaborative project has run into real problems . . . [and] the community staff have to go through a great deal . . . I want to get the acute unit strategy right by the end of this year. After that, I really want to tackle the local authority head on, on their own ground. I want to get into a major public relations strategy to fight theirs – which is, of course, highly elaborated.

But this was not the only response to the revived interest in municipal health care. One rich and powerful district, faced simultaneously with major financial cuts, a left-wing council and a highly active CHC, attempted to create a popular front in its pursuit of greater funding. Far from opposing local councillors' techniques of mass mobilization, the district reached out to embrace them. The politics of members and officers might differ but on this they were united. Some flavour of the methods and the strains in this strategy of alliance are captured in the following quotations:

> *DFD:* There have been big improvements in some areas in our political relations. Our relations with the CHC have gone up 1,000 per cent! A lot of time has gone into that . . . though our relations with region have gone right down.

> *CNA:* We have our politicians on it [DHA], but the standard of debate is high and the amount of political posturing is low. That has changed slightly because now we have a bigger percentage of people who want to toe the party line. We actually have members who are running to the press independently of the health authority – which never happened before. Also there's a bit of confusion as the trade union member is employed by the council in their health and environment committee – so it's a nice question as to whether she's asking questions as a member, or for her job. But, having said that, she's sophisticated and always keen to get us involved in prevention. Her arguments are always rational.

> *DGM:* Who's going to the public meeting on Thursday [on the district's strategy for managing the cuts]? The format is that myself and the chair and representatives from the CHC and the town council will speak; then it's thrown open to the floor. It would be nice if we had a selection of some officers. I want Jim [DPD] to come and Jean [DMO] will be coming along after attending the MAC. Are you coming, Brian [DFD]?

> *DFD:* I'm afraid I'm away but I will be sending one of my staff.

> *CNA:* That's very important. There'll be a lot of financial questions.

> *DFD:* If I fill it up with my staff, there'll be a lot of cheers every time general management is mentioned!

> *DGM:* The CHC has written to all the general managers to ask if they want to reserve seats.

## Conclusion

Local politics was, therefore, yet another powerful force which structured every district. If size, capital stock, population and the state of the local economy shaped every district health authority in their own distinctive fashion, so too did the local press, radio and television, the varying power and enthusiasm of voluntary groups, the state and organization of social services and the power and ideology of local politicians. General management, if it was to work, had to match local as well as national needs, had to satisfy local as well as national pressures.

# Headquarters' staff and structure

In this final chapter on district, we step back from the problems of the DGH and the giant Victorian mental hospital, retreat from the intricacies of local politics and social services and enter the bureaucratic sanctum itself – the headquarters' building where members met occasionally but the officers worked every day. In the first section of this chapter we tour district headquarters and inspect the new staff. In the second section, we examine the new management structures created in each district and the ways in which these were shaped by the diversity of local circumstance.

## The new leaders

Consider the DGMs first. Although the government had thrown such posts open to all applicants, most DGMs were appointed from within the NHS and most, in fact, came from its traditional administrative class. There were very few businessmen and just a handful of doctors and nurses. This in itself was a setback to the government's plans but, despite this, many new DGMs seem to have worked well enough. In the districts we examined, some more or less coherent form of teamwork and leadership had been established – although there were, certainly, stories of failures elsewhere. Not every new manager proved a success:

> *RPD:* The potential in Griffiths is certainly there – and the pitfalls. General managers have been given their head but the converse of that is that some general managers don't know how to use the freedom they've been given and a few are running amok!

In our study, at least, we came across no such disasters – at least among the DGMs. But if the DGMs we encountered were a relative success, they still varied markedly in their style and philosophy of leadership. Every new management team bore the influence of the DGM's personality, for there were many ways of running teams, some tender, some tough:

> *DGM:* The difficulty would be when I would have to say, 'Well, I'm sorry but that's gone beyond your powers'. Or whatever. I don't think it will honestly happen . . . We're actually in a situation where we've grown into an understanding that we've

got a role to play. Now that role isn't in small boxes away from one another. It's actually really a circle and everybody touches everybody else's fingers.

*CNA:* Griffiths works here because of the people and the open communication and me taking an active role. In the past nurses have been seen as a threat and neutralized. But now in this district, that's not the case. Here, we're encouraged to make our maximum contribution. It's the ability to sit down with the general manager and the senior nurses in a unit on a regular basis to sort out problems . . . Everyone contributes something different, but really we're working together.

*DGM:* I'm not authoritarian, but I don't suffer fools gladly!

*DPD:* I do find – which I shall tell her [DGM] when I have an appraisal – that I do feel up before the beak! I actually blush! It's a very physical thing. Jim [CNA] feels exactly the same. On the other hand, I do respect her. She's very straight and she doesn't bullshit.

*DNS:* Shirley [DGM] is not a woman to cross. Never tell her a lie! She'll accept the truth but if you lie – oh boy!

*INT:* You've worked with him [DGM] before.

*CNA:* Oh, yes, but working with someone who's an equal, it's a very different situation to working with somebody who has an absolute authority, or almost absolute authority over you . . . He still has a tendency – that's his personality, he'll not change that whatever job he does – you know he is an autocrat by nature. Albeit he sometimes tries to be a fairly benevolent autocrat . . . that's the most appropriate management style in the organization isn't it?

If the new leaders varied in the firmness with which they controlled their new teams, so too did their stress on formal statement and structure. In some districts there was a written summary of the district's new philosophy; in others there was not:

*CNA/Deputy DGM:* [Of the] two things [that] have concentrated our minds . . . the first is the district's mission statement. This says that we value our patients, value our staff, that we don't, won't, worry too much about local bureaucratic rules – if you can take a short cut, take it and we will back you.

*CNA:* The district hasn't got a formal statement of its philosophy. We've never had any discussion on this . . . I think it's, in practice, a very pluralistic sort of philosophy.

And, where some DGMs used formal structures quite heavily, others preferred to do most things through informal groups:

*DFD:* We haven't got a core management group and I don't believe we will . . . [instead] we've adopted a task-oriented approach – particular officers come together for particular issues. Where it becomes an overall concern, it goes to the DGM [district management group] . . . In the past, you had groups to look at an issue with representatives from every single group and you ended up with huge groups. We're certainly getting away from that. We're a lot more streamlined – though the new groups may bring in outsiders on a one off basis for a piece of advice.

Finally, there were differences in the speed with which DGMs moved and in their strategic sense. Some moved fast to implement Griffiths, others took their time:

DMO: Graham [DGM] thinks *long* – that's what I've learned from him. [Original emphasis] . . . He's taken the district a staggering distance in the last few years.

DFD: I don't know whether we're going fast or slow [in reorganizing structures]. I get the impression that some districts decided 'Bang!' and are just doing it. I'm for the middle road. You need the ability to adapt. It's certainly taken longer than I thought. Only now are we getting down to the nuts and bolts.

DMO: The structures are taking an enormously long time because Jim [DGM] keeps on sending them back. I expect the UGMs thought they could just produce one of those plans with little boxes dangling down on strings – they had another think coming! Jim wants tasks specified and he won't be satisfied until he's sure that the UGMs have got all the central tasks spelt out. Jobs have got to fit round real, necessary tasks.

## The headquarters' staff

DGMs therefore varied. So too did their headquarters' staff. As a new DGM assembled her staff on her very first day, what sort of prospect lay in front of her? Just who were her colleagues and what kind of team would they make? The prospect was not always appealing. Community medicine and nurse management, so it appeared, might be far from the only weak links. Indeed, in some districts there were problems with quite a few of the officers:

DGM: Coming into the health authority, I saw a lot of people who had come here to retire. They wanted an easy time – 'Nothing to tax you out there' – just joining for the last ten years of their career. Several of the chief officers were coming up to retirement and they didn't see the need to change anything. Just as long as everything was ticking over, why change?

Other districts might have higher overall standards, but even here there could still be many areas of difficulty. Major weaknesses could exist in any department. Although far more DGMs had been appointed from the ranks of the old administrators than from any other group, not every senior administrator was seen as possessing managerial gifts:

DCh: I formed the view within five minutes that the administrator wasn't up to the job. A born ditherer. The old chair showed me some letters that Sheila [administrator] had given him to sign. I said, 'I wouldn't sign one of those. They're all rubbish!'

Likewise, although staff development was now in vogue and personnel directors were on the up and up, some had doubts about their ability to do all that was now asked of them:

INT: Personnel used to be very low status.
DPD: Yes, it first took off in 74 and then 84 gave it a major boost . . . Griffiths though is going to have to combine administration and personnel a bit because managers can't divorce themselves from the staff for which they're responsible.

UGMs are going to have to learn new techniques in staff management . . . One of the things Bob [DGM] is very keen on here is staff appraisal. We're having a session at the next board meeting on management development. This is something with which the NHS is totally unfamiliar. But it's very tricky. An operator has to be very skilled to avoid confrontation . . . I mugged up all the old texts and then confronted Bob with the various techniques – he got quite a shock!

*DPD:* We [personnel] are expanding in all directions but we're having to retain our costs within overall management costs and therefore there are problems. In fact, stress is becoming a problem – and that's the last thing you want in a personnel department!

Financial managers, another key priority under the new arrangements, also had serious problems. Treasurers – as they had been called – had not been particularly powerful in the past:

*DFD:* My view is that finance is integral to the management task. The traditional NHS view is that treasurers just keep the books and tell you when you've overspent! I found it unbelievable when I came here from a local authority job. In local authorities – of course it varies – but the treasurer is high status because of the rates. In the NHS, the treasurer was low status.

Now, however, that status had radically changed. But, given the previous neglect, although some districts had impressive financial leadership, elsewhere there might be doubts. Was the treasurer actually up to the mark? Some were, others were not. Consider those comments from three separate districts:

*DGM:* Quite frankly, he [finance director] isn't up to it yet. The job's beyond him at the moment.

*DGM:* What we have here is a treasurer and not a finance director – with all that that implies in the loss of creative thinking . . . We've papered over the cracks. He has improved, but there's still a very heavy element of book keeping in his work.

*CNA:* The financial information in this district is poor; in fact, very weak. We've not got the staff and the staff we have got are not appropriately qualified. The financial information in X district, where I was before, was very different; the quality of the information was much better.

Getting good managers had, therefore, proved hard. Some districts turned instead to hybrid roles. Others to outsiders as the government had urged health authorities. In both cases, there were problems:

*DFD:* Posts haven't been a problem so far – but they will be. A lot of people are going for unit accountants and upping grades to do it. I'm not convinced that there are the people there to fill them. Our long-term aim is to educate UGMs to take a more financial role.

*DCh:* Ministers hoped that we could bring in outside business people. We had forty or fifty people apply for the DGM's post – a high proportion of whom were outsiders. Almost all of them were people who in some way were in difficulty. It was a way out rather than a positive choice. Their firm had been shut down; it had been amalgamated; or they were at the end of their contract. I concluded that the perception of the NHS in business is that it is grossly inefficient and badly managed. All my friends say this. It's partly true, but a lot of it is very unfair – but it's what they think. As a result, a very ambitious manager who went into the NHS would have serious re-entry problems into the private sector. They'd look at his CV and say, 'Why did he do that? He must be no good.' That's one of the reasons we got so few good outside applicants.

Even where good outsiders could be obtained, they might still need lengthy training in the appropriate NHS skills – as the following views on an external finance director indicate:

*DGM:* She [ex-finance director] did a super job. She created lots of important new initiatives . . . I learnt a lot from her . . . I have to say, though, that she was not strong on implementation. She was more an ideas woman.

*CNA:* She didn't understand NHS financing. All the billing in the units was a mess. They hadn't paid the nursing school invoices for six months and they weren't actually paid until April 1st. So nurse education actually began the financial year with an overspend!

## The chairman

If the quality of the officers shaped every district's structure, so too did that of its chairman. Their new powers were fundamental. Appointed first in the new management structures, it was chairmen who played the key role in selecting the new DGMs. But, just as officers varied dramatically, so did chairmen. One summarized his job like this:

*DCh.* I'm a busy chap. So it's no good me trying to know all the details. So, by temperament and necessity, when I have little heart to hearts with the DGM, I say, 'Your job is to run the district machine, while I chair the health authority, appoint the members and manage the relations with ministers and MPs. You keep out of that – that's what I do! Other things we do together.' I expect to be consulted on the agenda and strategy and I'm obviously informed if anything goes wrong. I have a weekly meeting with the DGM and we talk about where things are going and the financial and service strategy. That's the most effective thing I do. It's just an informal natter. All reports come to me in their first draft. It's not my prerogative to alter them. If I think they're plainly wrong, I do – but I never censor them. I also say what I don't understand – what doesn't make sense. I also take charge of things that are of local political interest, like the recent hospital closure. Otherwise – for example, the trouble on the paediatric ward at the Royal – I don't know what it is and I don't very much care! I just deal with the major things – the major sites and the major finance.

Such a description might seem to fit some ideal norm for the new style of chairman. But, in fact, there was no such thing as a typical district chair. Another chair might play a useful role but be subordinate to a powerful DGM. Yet another be a laughing stock throughout the district. Some might involve themselves in national organizations. Others ignored all that and stuck close to their own turf:

*DFD:* There's no doubt about who rules this district – and it ain't the members! The chairman's a sweetie but Jim [DGM] is the puppet master!

*DGM:* The chairman wants to be kept informed but he doesn't do anything when he is. So it's all appearance. He exasperates everybody because he's so egocentric and stand offish. He doesn't let anyone near him.

*DNS:* The chairman is hopeless. He waves his arms about and threatens to walk out. He's not exactly dynamic. It's worth going to see him for a laugh. His behaviour is very funny. (*pause*) He's just been reappointed.

*DMO:* I've learned a staggering amount about how to manage a health authority meeting from Shirley [DGM]. And the way she manages the chairman – he's an absurd man, no, absurd is too kind – it's an absolute joy to watch. Though I'm sure some of Shirley's problems with the authority are due to lack of support from the chairman.

*DCh:* I don't see the other chairs very much. I went to one of those NAHA meetings and thought, 'Never, never, never again'! They don't grab me!

The effects of such diversity were more important than variation in some of the other senior management positions. It might be hard to attract officers with business experience, but it was much easier to get a chairman with such qualifications. Besides, although the role of chairman was merely part-time, some turned it into a full-time post, soaking themselves in the life of the authority and playing a major role in its direction. One such provided the glue that held the district together, mediating between a powerful DGM and other talents in the authority and providing a particular philosophy of management:

*DCh:* When I became chairman in 1981, I recommended, with my business background, that there shouldn't be an elderly chairman like myself, that what was needed was a lively executive – but the minister didn't listen, they never do! Nevertheless, we got consensus management working very well indeed and when they decided to implement a chief executive structure, we moved to the 'three-legged stool' [general management, nursing and medicine].

There were other ways besides the philosophy of management for a chairman to be busy. A key element in the role of the fully active chair was deep involvement with the life of the locality, with the fêtes, the pressure groups and the staff of every kind:

*DGM:* We now have a young chair who is just so totally committed to the job – the daughter of Lord Grimsby. She's come in and she's looked and she's looked thoroughly and gained the respect of members. She puts in a huge amount of time. On Saturdays and Sundays she attends all kinds of things. She's also on all kinds of national committees [X, Y and Z] and has close links to the Tory party. She's a very remarkable woman . . . She's so enthusiastic. We've prepared a slide talk for her and she goes round the district trying to persuade everyone that they're just one part of the big picture.

At the extreme, the fully active chair could be centrally involved in the daily life of district management, working closely alongside the DGM, as in the following district:

*DCh:* I attend the executive board meetings – which I don't think many chairmen do – as I need to find out what they're up to! Otherwise, it'll all go on behind my back! This job is supposed to be one and a half days a week. In fact, it's six days a week.

*DGM:* I find the chairman very helpful and supportive. Graham [RGM] tells me he interferes too much but I think it's a good fault and I'm very glad to have his support and involvement. In fact, I wouldn't have been so keen to have done the job had I not known the chairman very well. He's got an ideal background. He's familiar with state organizations, he knows something about health and he understands finance.

In short, the role and quality of chairmen varied. Like directors of finance and personnel, like general managers too, there was enormous local diversity; a diversity which matched the huge range of variation that was found in every other aspect of a district's life.

## Local circumstances, local structures

Up until now, we have focused on the many ways in which districts might vary. In the final part of this chapter we examine some of the consequences of this variation for Griffiths. The first task for the new DGM was the creation of a new formal structure. Griffiths might be flexible, but a new organization needed a new plan, an organizational chart which laid out in some simple form the new hierarchy and division of labour. The capital stock had to be divided into new management units; the new management staff – with all their widely varying competence – had to be given new roles.

However, although all the headquarters' staff now fell under a single line of command, DGMs could not simply rule by fiat. The new structure had, ideally, to enlist the enthusiasm and support of the new management team; it depended on complex negotiations with the team, on their point of view as well as the DGM's. And, if the subordinate managers could shape the new structures, so too could the health authority members and the management tiers that lay above district. The DHSS and the regions wished to ensure that every district implemented general management; the locality wanted to check that it did so in a way that met local needs. There was also the legacy of the previous management team and, as in everything else the huge influence of each district's size and capital stock. Each of these factors is considered in the sections which follow.

## Official approval

If members were typically weak, they none the less varied like everything else. Some sided with groups who were threatened by the new structures. Some were even encouraged to intervene by the new managers. In one district, the health authority had a Griffiths sub-committee with considerable formal power over the new management structure. One of the consequences had been a long delay in deciding what to do about nursing advice. A DNS had filled the post temporarily while the members watched her work and decided whether a post at district was really necessary:

> DGM: It was the authority who were not convinced of the need for a CNA and some of that is down to – if you like – the low profile that nursing has had in this district. And the fact that few reports were put [in the past] to the members . . . One certainly gets the impression that members just didn't understand what a CNA would do . . . They had difficulty from their previous experience in seeing a high profile, pro-active individual, influencing them and me and having a role to play in the running of the district . . . It was always going to be some time before we progressed this, so that the members could see a different type of individual. But there's an involvement there [in the new CNA – previously the acting CNA]. There's an individual who puts her foot down – and that's not just to test the water, I mean that's actually to say that, 'We're not going down there!' It's somebody that's walking the patch. She walks the patch much more than I do – and I walk it a lot. We keep on passing each other in the car!

But, of course, most members were weak. Regions, however, possessed more power over the new district structures. Where there were disagreements, district managers could be sent away to think again:

> DGM: We were the first [in this region] to submit our plans and the last to be accepted! As a result, though I would ideally have gone to advertise in October, we hadn't got the green light. In fact, the UGM posts weren't advertised until May or June.

Again, take nursing as an example of what regional intervention might mean and the different ways in which it might affect the new structures. Within England, there was no central line on the provision of professional nursing advice at regional or district level. The Department issued circulars and requested information, but mostly did not intervene. There had to be a mechanism for such advice, but how this was done was left to the managers concerned:

> INT: How has the recent letter from the Minister about the DMO affected you?
> RM: Which one? We get so many! Circulars, huh! . . . There's been no pressure from the Department over the RNO [who had been removed]; only from the RCN. Insofar as there was any pressure from DHSS, it was just asking for explanations. It was nothing.

As a result, the matter was left to both district and region to decide:

> CNA: In the RGM's letter to the DGM there was quite a bit about the CNA's role – although some important issues were omitted. For example, I don't know whether I will be involved in the appointment of senior nurses . . . It's based on a letter from DHSS which raises a number of important questions about the CNA's role, about

appointments, disciplinary procedures and so forth. So I want to have a chat with Jim [DGM] before he answers it.

*RNO:* This is the only region where we've insisted that there be a nurse at a senior level in every district . . . X district have got a proposed structure with a UGM who's a nurse offering professional advice at district. I will not allow this in this region! [In this region one or two districts eventually got away with advice based at unit.]

*RPD:* At a regional level, we haven't had any policy as regards nursing management.

*RGM:* In my region, we start off from a zero base. I'm fed up with the professions banging the drum. In some districts, there's no need for a DMO or a DNO; in others there is. It all depends on the needs of the district. If your nursing advisory committee has got it right, there's no absolute need for a DNO. The key thing is to get things done.

*CNA:* I had another look at Griffiths the other day. . . . I was very keen on it at first! . . . [but] . . . in this region, the RGM and the chair tried to wipe nurses off all the boards. I decided they weren't going to get rid of me, because I think I've got a very good track record and the nurses here are very good . . . When the DGM was appointed and suggested his new structures, the fights began . . . The RGM shouted down the corridor to him, 'Get rid of her!' He wanted me to go because he saw me as a powerful leader. I got hold of some of the documents. They wanted to wipe nurses off everything . . . I think they thought nurses would be a push over . . . Some of the senior nurses were having their offices and secretaries taken away from them – it was terrible – and told to look for another job . . . [Someone who had been on the RHA] told me that in 1974, the administrators had bitterly resented nurses being added as part of the team. I never had that feeling myself, but this is what she said . . . [When they failed to abolish all the CNO posts] the RGM sent a letter to all the DGMs asking for CNO's salaries to be reduced as their responsibilities were less than other executive team members.

Regions, then, could exert real power – and not just over nursing. So one crucial thing that the new DGMs faced when they started to implement Griffiths was the views, not just of Griffiths or the NHS management board, but of the new RGM, the RFD, the RPD, the RNO and all the other officers of the regional board; some powerful, some weak, some interested, some not. But, of course, there were many other factors which went into the making of the new district structures.

## The power of the clinical trades: a case-study of nursing

The new structures were not simply selected by management and members; they could also be shaped by the struggle with the clinical trades. Doctors exerted a powerful influence on the new organizational charts. Even nurses still had the power to fight back. Indeed all the management trades could exert an important influence upon the new structures. Before the new DGMs could take their plans to members and region for official approval, there was lengthy negotiation with personnel, finance, nursing, medicine and so forth.

Nurses had the reputation of being the weakest members of the old district management team and were the group that suffered most in the Griffiths reorganization. Some, however, played their own, independent role in the creation of the new structures. Not every CNO offered successful resistance. Many took early retirement. But there were others who were powerful enough – or held in sufficient esteem by the new general managers – to choose the job that they wanted, turning down some, selecting others:

> CNA: I was offered a hybrid role of personnel director and chief nurse advisor . . . but [I turned it down] . . . I didn't think they'd thought it through. It was a change for change's sake. And I also felt it would harm nursing. Two of the senior nurses here tried to persuade me to take it on, saying it would enhance nursing's power. But I felt it would actually diminish it because it would distract me from the development of nursing, from building it up – and that's a big enough job by itself.

Even where a nursing post at district had been abolished and advice was now given from unit level, the person selected could still have some influence upon the structure – just to be wanted gave some measure of power:

> CNA/DNE: She [DGM] feels very strongly that the DNE should be accountable to the director of personnel and I feel very strongly that they shouldn't be . . . Although I think nurse education has to be part of the district training strategy, it's not the be all and end all of it, because we do have a role regionally and nationally . . . I almost said, 'If that's your view, I will have to look for an option out' and because I expressed it so strongly it was a compromise in the end.

Such personal negotiation was not the only option for those who disliked their place in the new structure. All kinds of tactics might be tried. Some nurses ignored the new rules, downed tools, appealed to the members, sought out the press, got aid from their professional network or lobbied MPs and peers:

> CNA: Region tried to divest the RNO of all her support staff but she's gradually getting them back again. Indeed, at one stage, region tried to abolish the RNO post entirely. All the CNAs were told to send their manpower reports to someone else at region – and not the RNO. However, we all sent her a spare copy.

> CNA: We won through here because we simply withdrew from committees until the DGM discovered the organization couldn't do without us. It all started with a dispute over casualty. We insisted that only a registered nurse could have responsibility for individual patients. There are one or two places here that have given that responsibility to enrolled nurses. He complained that we were interfering in managerial decisions. So we withdrew and eventually he had to come and ask us to take part in things once more.

> DNS: I was quite prepared, if necessary, to take this to the point where I would bring it into the public arena and make it a political thing. I hoped I wouldn't have to do that, so what I did first of all, I saw the members for the hospital, met up with them and put it to them, 'Look, this is what is planned. In our heart of hearts, I know this is wrong and I will fight it tooth and nail . . .' I didn't have to say it too openly, but I did hint fairly broadly that we would fight it to the bitter end.

> CNA: I wrote out my own job description and gave it to the other CNOs to help

them. And the CNO from X district, who had been told to go, read it out at a health authority meeting and the authority told the DGM that that's what they wanted for their nurses too. So they told him to rewrite the structure. And, gradually, apart from Y, the CNOs got back.

*CNA:* I had the press after me and the RGM rang up and said, 'I'm fed up with reporters hanging around me asking about your job. You've no right to do this.' I said, 'I have every right. It's a democratic country and I have every right to defend myself and my profession' . . . I went to the Lords with some very good nurses from A . . . Baroness Oswestry told me the government was very worried about the RCN's campaign . . . I saw Lord Thurso too.

There were, therefore, a number of tactics by which officers could seek to modify the plans of the new general management. However, only the most powerful CNAs could risk such confrontation. For some DGMs, public opposition – or even backstage manoeuvring to that end – was quite beyond the pale:

*DGM:* What put the seal on it [the removal of the CNO] was a DHA meeting. Chris [old CNO] was away at a conference, so a DNS was acting up. We'd agreed that all the budgets would be reduced by 1 per cent. Chris had gone along with it grudgingly. At the DHA meeting we were about to reach a resolution when the nurse member asked a question and the DNS blurted out that Chris had told her to say that, if the nursing budget was reduced, patients would be at risk. It's the only time in my life that I've changed colour! Subsequent enquiries showed that the nurse member had been set up.

*INT:* Isn't this quite common?

*DGM:* I've never seen it before. It's just not acceptable.

*CNA (speaking at a local management conference):* The fact that the CNA can go to the DHA may be true but it's so threatening to the DGM that it isn't a weapon one would ever want to use.

*DGM:* You make it sound like a nuclear weapon! (*loud laughter*)

The audience might laugh but the facts were real enough. The clinical managers had the formal right to oppose district policy at DHA meetings, if they felt this was required on clinical grounds. But going to the authority on a fundamental matter was a Doomsday strategy which only a few could use without fear of annihilation. None the less, for all their weakness, nurse managers were not wholly without power. Nor, too, were their fellow officers. Structures, therefore, were not simply imposed. They also depended on careful, internal negotiation.

## Size, capital stock and structure

Since capital, more than any other factor, shaped the nature and direction of districts, the way it was distributed had a huge impact on the new management structures. One key factor which shaped the extent of devolution was simple geographical size. A vast rural district whose population and institutions were very widely scattered had good reason to decentralize some key functions. The rationale might be less clear in a small, closely packed and wholly urban district where most services were concentrated on the same site. Such factors would operate quite independently of unit structure. The first quotation below is taken from a vast district with a consequent policy of massive devolution – but which contained just the one unit; the district was the unit. The second came from an urban district which was now divided into three units but which still kept some key management functions at the centre:

DGM: It [district] is a hundred miles long and fifty miles wide . . . The main problem here is communication . . . We've just put in our own district phone system so that all calls will be local. Before that every time you phoned a hospital – and we've got a good many here, every call was a trunk call! . . . I thought it was nonsense the way we were organized [into three units]. We were so split up I went for a single unit . . . There are three separate counties you know – or there were in the past – and they think of themselves still like that and we've got to break that . . . [but] you can't plan from the centre in this district . . . I decided that the best way forward was to identify centres of population around hospitals and then to integrate the services there even closer. Each of these would have a locality manager – each of these centres of population around each hospital. So we ended up with twelve locality managers in all.

DFD: We're not delegating paymaster responsibility to units. Instead, we're proposing to retain the management accounting function. We're not going for unit accountants. There's no point because of their small size and physical location – the fact, for example, that the acute unit is just across the road.

So the size of a district and the distribution of its capital stock could shape the extent of devolution quite independently of structure. But units were still of fundamental concern to the reorganized NHS. When units had been created in 1982, there was a powerful feeling in Whitehall that many districts had handled the matter badly. The new instructions from the top were to reduce the number of units into which each district was divided and simultaneously to devolve far more real power to those units. However, not every district had carried out the new central policy of reducing their number, while some still excluded the heads of the units, the UGMs, from the new district management teams. Such reluctance to change was strongly criticized in some quarters:

ML: Structures which don't have the UGMs at the top table are very hard to explain.

Such apparent opposition to ministerial wishes had several different causes. One reason was simply a desire to minimize change:

INT: Why have you retained the same number of units?
DGM: Idleness! It was! Actually, we'd only recently set up the structure and I felt very reluctant to make changes for change's sake. Our unit management groups were only just beginning to work – after two years! I didn't want to change things just when they'd really got going. I wanted to give them a chance to do well.

So change could be a problem in creating new units. So too was the overall size of the district. A small district could more readily have a small number of units; just two or three, for example. A reduction to such numbers might potentially save administrative costs and there were huge central pressures on districts to actually save money through management reorganization. On the other hand, such a move could create serious tensions. Jobs might be lost; those who were once equal members of the same trade might now be forced to compete for the same job knowing that one would become master over the other; different branches of the same trade might enter into rivalry. Consider the problems that emerged in the nursing service when districts reduced the numbers of their units:

> CNA: There are only going to be two units and we've got four DNSs, so they need treating very carefully. I've just heard on the phone that one of them is very anxious and is causing a lot of trouble in her unit.

> DCh: We're cutting our units from four to two . . . One of them is acute services; the other is a spread of things. On the acute side, there'll be a unit management board with a DNS on it but she'll be under the UGM instead of the old consensus management. It's very straightforward. The one difficulty, however, is the merging of obstetrics and midwifery – that's a real problem, a source of real tension. The other unit is more generally a problem. For management to keep within budget, we can't afford – financially or practically – a situation in which the four or five divisions within the new unit will each have a separate administrator, a separate DNS and so forth. Therefore, we're going to appoint service managers and they may come from any of the occupations. If it's a nurse, she'll still be a nurse, so she'll be two things – so we won't appoint a DNS under her. Where they are not a nurse, well, almost certainly but not absolutely certainly, we'll appoint a DNS. It rather depends on who comes forward.

Such a reduction in the number of units could also produce a major clash between managerial and professional responsibilities. Consider an example from a third district:

> CNA: Unfortunately what has happened is that – and I've been arguing this but I haven't won this one – with the appointment of the DNS on the acute unit, midwifery was subsumed under it. The director of midwifery services is responsible to the director of nursing services, acute – and that to me is quite wrong . . . and what of course has highlighted it and made it critical that we break that down is that we have had a professional disciplinary problem and, of course, the DNS was quite annoyed to find that she had no role at all to play in this. I mean what it amounts to is that you've got a nominal manager there who knows nothing about the service and who can't accept the professional responsibility either.

Thus, the general manager of a small district faced contrasting pressures when constructing a new structure. Size and ease of administration conflicted with the demands from the old managerial and professional staff. Those who managed large districts faced somewhat different dilemmas. Districts that stayed with a large number of units were released from some problems. There was more managerial work for the members of different trades and thus less immediate pressure to amalgamate different jobs. On the other hand, they might face severe problems of representation. A very large district with a big population and a large number of services might have created six, seven, even eight sizable units in 1982. But, if some of these were now to be amalgamated, the resulting bodies could be very unwieldy. On the other hand, if the old structures were retained, what would happen to the position of the new UGMs? Could a district executive board which included all the district officers as well as the seven or eight UGMs be a serious decision-making body? Committees with more than six or seven members were often clumsy affairs.

> *CNA (large teaching district):* When we looked at units, there was a strong case for amalgamating all the units in the city [there were four based on five separate hospitals] because the consultants are interchangeable – but then the size would be far too big. It would be a mini-district all by itself. We had a dilemma. Did we go for macro-units – which would be too big. Or did we stay with the units we had – which would mean excluding UGMs from the board – as that would be too big?

Different districts resolved these pressures in different ways. But whatever was eventually decided, the new structures were powerfully shaped by the welter of local factors, by the size of the district, by the capital stock, by the often contradictory needs of both the old and the new managers, as well as by ministers, regions, members and the power of the clinical trades. Thus, as they sketched out their provisional organizational charts, DGMs were pulled in one direction after another by a host of local and national pressures. They were also, as we shall now see, fundamentally influenced by the quality of the team – and of the structures– which they inherited from the past.

## The old team and the new

The local implementation of Griffiths was necessarily shaped by the old district management team, by its relative success or failure, by the extent to which the old members were still available for service, by the previous local attempts at reform. In some districts, for example, Griffiths-style innovations were under way well before 1984 – an experience which, in different ways, shaped Griffiths's reception:

> *DGM:* In X district, where I was DNO, we had a very strong management team and – although it's hackneyed to say it – we'd all got special responsibilities. So I was in charge, not just of nursing but also of the psychiatric side and, likewise, the mental handicap side. I started off a major project – which ended up involving three districts – and I got a new building into commission in under a year! Unheard of! . . . So, in a way, I was a general manager already.

> *CNA:* I was fortunate in coming to a district where the officers have genuinely been given a mandate to be entrepreneurs. Moreover, in this district – and indeed in this region, the change to Griffiths-style management came very early. We had it up and running in 1983.

> *DFD:* We've got ward budgets now in most units. We've come a long way in the

last few years. I introduced the idea before Patients First . . . and we had one or two administrators who were very keen . . . We started with separate budget books in the first year – 82 – for each hospital. So really it was happening here anyway . . . It had been very centralist but way before Griffiths we were into devolution, into making people responsible for their budgets and giving them virement policies so that overspending was carried forward – giving them a total allocation of cash, rather than holding them to individual budgets. You can do what you like within the budget which is revolutionary for the NHS – but I kill them if it gets out of control! . . . Forty years of overspending at the infirmary was transformed over three months to being bang on.

*CNA:* I thought Frank [DA] left a real balls up. He implemented Griffiths before its time. In 82, for example, the units were given almost complete independence. He made all the nursing staff responsible to the DNSs – but the CNO wasn't responsible *for* the DNSs. Typical! [Original emphasis]

*CNA:* Our health authority didn't really want Griffiths. When we started in 82, we were overspent by £2 million, care was in a mess and there was no plan. By 84, it was all sorted out. We did a huge amount of work. I've never worked with people who *worked* so hard – fourteen hours a day. We got all the budgets down to the wards. So really we didn't want Griffiths. (Original emphasis)

The new team was also moulded by the old. There was a huge difference between districts in which the DMT had worked well together and those where it had not. There was also a major difference between districts in which the officers had survived largely intact and those where key players had gone off to new jobs. Consider three strongly contrasted circumstances in which a new team and its leader was created. In one district, the old team had disintegrated, the key players departed and new managers were brought in, some of whom had little time for those few who had remained:

*DMO:* District's not as much fun as it was. I really used to enjoy DMT. We were much more social. With ten of us on the board now it makes it much more difficult. And there's only two of us left from the original DMT.

*DFD:* The reality is we have a board within a board. The DGM, the two UGMs and me meet on a clandestine basis! The other guys are nice guys but they don't input a damn thing. I don't believe anybody has got the right to a place on the board as a matter of course.

At the other extreme, was a district where the previous and relatively successful DMT had remained largely intact. Indeed, it had exerted a powerful collective influence on the new structures that emerged. As a result, powerful elements of the old consensus management had been retained within the new team:

*DCh:* I spent a long time [when I was first appointed] – in fact two months, trying to get to know the chief officers and some of the key doctors . . . It did seem to me very clear that the concept of chief officers was the right one and that they [the officers] with one exception were really rather good . . . I suggested Alf [a doctor] for DGM and the chief officers said en bloc that none of them would apply for the post if Alf did – but that they'd all apply en bloc if Sheila put in for it!

*CNA:* There's a very strong feeling of being a team here. We get on with each other. When we knew that Alf was interested in becoming the DGM, several of us [on the DMT] pushed quite hard for him . . . We knew that he wasn't a manager – it's management by common sense, not trained management – but we thought, we'd had that and he'd have some chance of influencing his colleagues.

*INT:* How does it compare with the old DMT?

*CNA:* It's very difficult to say without taking individuals into account. Sheila was a procrastinator beyond belief but she's gone now . . . She wasn't bad at analysing situations – just at taking decisions in case she was wrong . . . My authority hasn't really changed . . . Alf's style is, 'You're being paid, get on with it. Tell me if there are any problems.' The DNSs are still accountable to me – but now they're accountable also to the UGMs. The real change now is that we have a leader at district and unit level. But we've not changed anything else particularly. We've not changed things simply for the sake of change. Only if we think they're not performing. I'd delegated budgets to DNSs before general management came in. They only come to me about them if they've got a problem. You don't need to hold a budget to influence people. My planning nurse keeps me informed along with my personnel nurse. The team is much better than it was. It's just a personality thing . . . Griffiths has brought benefits. There is one person to whom I can go if I'm out of kilter with the other officers. Before I had to try and convert them in a meeting or one by one. Now I can go straight to Alf. I've used this on a couple of occasions.

In this second type of district, something of the structure and powers of the old functional management had been retained. However, there was one radical difference from the past – and one crucial resemblance to the district just mentioned where the old DMT had been swept to one side. Here too there was now a kitchen cabinet. Behind the new management committee, which differed little from the old DMT in its membership, lay a close alliance of the chair and the new DGM. This duumvirate always brought matters to the weekly meetings of the committee for their approval, but it was they who, in the end, held the power. Here, too, there were now leaders.

A third type stood between these two poles. Where the old DMTs had had successful administrators, they were often appointed as new DGMs; so here, although there might well have been radical change, there was strong continuity too. Some powerful administrators had, in fact, already acted almost as if they were DGMs. The following quotations come from three separate districts:

*DNS:* Jeff's appointment as DGM has made no difference to things. He runs the district just as he did when he was district administrator!

*INT:* What sort of difference has Ian [DGM] made?

*CNA:* When he arrived [as administrator] he came with an aura! People where he was before said, 'The big, bad Ian Hamilton!' The joke later was, 'He wrote Griffiths!' . . . What impressed me was the way that, from the beginning, he challenged the autonomy of medical staff.

*DCh:* Our administrator was a very dominant person. So we had a DGM *de facto* if not *de jure* [who then became DGM].

Griffiths, then, was flexible. Districts could be ruled in different ways. No doubt there were many other types of structure besides the few we have sketched here; and no structure was stable. As managers died, moved on or retired, so structures changed. By the end of our study, four out of our seven main districts had experienced fundamental staff change. The DGMs left and so too did three UGMs, one chairman, and one finance director. And, as they left, so too did particular styles of leadership, coalitions and inner cabinets. Structure was essential but change was permanent.

## Conclusion

The NHS, then, was a local as much as a national affair. Each district was embedded simultaneously within a distinct geographical area and within a hierarchical organization that stretched up to the Secretary of State. And, just as it was firmly embedded in the local economy and in local politics, so it was locally embodied in poor law and cottage hospitals, or in a brand new DGH. That embodiment also took a more human form. The management teams, charged with matching the diversity of local circumstance to the new methods of organization, could vary quite as much as the quality of the architecture or the size of the population. If Griffiths was to succeed, it was here, in the localities, in districts and units, that its success or failure would be measured.

Of course, in bending to local context, Griffiths was doing no more than every previous reorganization. Whatever the formal national structures, the NHS had always necessarily allowed considerable local variation in the way things were actually run. What made Griffiths different was that its model of management tried, quite explicitly, to cater to local circumstance. Indeed, it made a positive virtue out of flexibility. It urged general managers to cut their coats with the cloth that was actually available, to create individual structures that matched each district's history, staff, size, population and capital stock. Here, then, there appeared at least some initial success.

But Griffiths was not simply a matter of structures. It was also – and just as fundamentally – about a new set of management powers and a new set of organizational goals. Cost and quality were the slogans on the banners it waved. Delegation, performance monitoring and a single overarching chain of command were the means it proposed to these ends. But, in health care, these are difficult goals to achieve. General management might be flexible but was it wise and powerful enough to run its huge and diverse empire – its vast rural districts, imperious medical schools and downtrodden, inner-city areas – with an efficiency, humanity and effectiveness that had never been accomplished before? In the final part of this book, we evaluate Griffiths, presenting both managers' views and our own.

# PART 5    GENERAL MANAGEMENT
## ASSESSED

# 10   Money and power .

When asked if the French Revolution had been a success, Chou En-Lai answered that it was still too early to say. Any evaluation of Griffiths is bound to be preliminary. But something must be said all the same. In the final part of this book we try to do six things: to assess how far the concrete reality of Griffiths actually matched the theory of general management; to examine how far the much vaunted devolution of power had really taken place; to consider whether the new leaders had sufficient power to enable them to lead; and sufficient information to enable them to lead wisely; to appraise the further reforms proposed in 1989 – reforms which were much closer to the pure model of general management than the tentative steps first introduced in 1984; and, finally to consider some intrinsic problems with the general management model.

We begin with a close examination of the way in which Griffiths was fundamentally a compromise; a new model of management which nevertheless made many striking concessions to traditional methods of organizing health care. The first part of this chapter considers the pure theory of general management, the remainder describes one of Griffiths's most basic deviations. As we shall see, the NHS might, at last, have leaders but, to the doctrinally pure at heart, they remained trapped within inflexible hierarchies and still subject to the massive countervailing power of medical syndicalism.

## General management theory and public services

Until now, we have treated 'Griffiths' and 'general management' as synonymous. The reality is rather different. While Griffiths drew deeply on the doctrines of general management theory, his report was also – and just as profoundly – a compromise with many decades, even centuries, of traditional health service administration. Such compromise is not surprising. Western medicine may be, more or less, international but health care systems are not. Though there is much that each now has in common, each national system is still heavily shaped by the past, by that unique mix of local experience that renders one country so different from another. The service that each country offers its citizens thus consists of a mixture of ancient institutions and venerable occupations combined, in a highly complex way, with new modifications and fresh growths. The historian, Charles Webster, has commented on the deep roots the NHS already had when it was first created in 1948:

> Although widely portrayed as a revolutionary departure, the National Health Service as a mechanism was in most respects evolutionary, or even traditional. For instance, although originally conceived as a unified structure, the service was effectively split into three distinct component parts coinciding with the three nuclei around which health care institutions had aggregated in the course of the previous century. Health services provided at public cost were also of venerable origin, having their source in the mechanisms evolved for poor relief in the sixteenth century. Finally, state-administered compulsory national health insurance was established in 1911 as a replacement for a variety of earlier contributory medical schemes.[1]

Griffiths, then, was obliged to build on the past. In doing so, it omitted one key feature of the modern general management creed – competition. The principles of general management had been developed primarily in the private sector and for the sale of goods – not for complex personal services such as health care. None the less, a few general management theorists had, for many decades, looked wistfully upon the public sector. Concrete applications might still lie in the business world, but they saw little reason why much the same principles might not be applied – just as fruitfully – to national and local government. In the quotation below, Peter Drucker, businessmen's favourite writer on general management, considers its relevance to services such as health care:

> The second kind of service institution is exemplified by schools, universities and hospitals. Most of the service staffs within business organizations belong here too . . . Its performance is crucial to modern developed society . . . Customers of this kind of service institution are not really customers. They are more like taxpayers. They pay for the service institution whether they want to or not, out of taxes, levies such as compulsory insurance, or overhead allocations. The products of these institutions do not supply a want. They supply a need. Schools, hospitals and the typical service staff in business supply what everybody should have, ought to have, must have, because it is 'good for them', or good for society . . . [Such] institutions . . . need a system like Oskar Lange's socialist competition. The objective – the overall mission – must be general for this kind of service institution. There must be minimum standards of performance and results. But for the sake of performance, it is highly desirable that they should have managerial autonomy and not be run by government, even if they are supervised and regulated by it. There should also be a fair amount of consumer choice between different ways of accomplishing the basic mission, between different priorities and different methods. There should also be enough competition for these institutions to hold themselves to performance standards . . . What the service institutions need is not better people. They need people who do the management job systematically and who focus themselves and their institution purposefully on performance and results. They do need efficiency – that is, control of costs – but above all they need effectiveness – emphasis on the right

results. Few service institutions today suffer from having too few administrators. Most of them are overadministered and suffer from a surplus of procedures, organization charts and management techniques. What we have to learn is to manage service institutions for performance. This may well be the most important management task in this century.[2]

As is immediately obvious, the 1984 NHS did not fit this doctrine at all. Griffiths might have been a revolution yet, instead of autonomy, the government still ran the service. And, instead of competition, there was only one source of provision. General management might have been introduced but the NHS remained a national monopoly, the single supplier of health care to the bulk of the population. Thus, some managers had serious doubts about the type of general management that Griffiths had now introduced. In this, and the next chapter, we consider the criticisms that they made. Once again, our analysis takes the form of a collage.

## Politicians' whims, Whitehall's stranglehold

Most managers' suspicions centred around government, though some still had some praise for the changes at the centre:

> *DGM:* The injection to the centre of people from the outside has changed DHSS a bit. There's more direction, a more determined level of activity. At one time, DHSS just told you to push off. The new boys are much more street-wise than most DHSS officials.

Despite this, there was also a widespread feeling that politicians and civil servants could simply never be trusted. Politicians' language was too often slippery and at odds with the reality of what was actually occurring. Their stress was on public relations, not on hard organizational truth:

> *RGM:* As for the annual report the government puts out on the NHS it's a scandal. Complete rubbish! What does all that data mean?

> *CNA:* Have you seen that video with Fowler [the Secretary of State] where he says [Griffiths] is not a reorganization at all! This is downright dishonesty! I've lost faith in him.

For most managers such matters were trivial – if symptomatic. Far more crucial, so they felt, was the way Whitehall was driven, not by the long-term needs of the NHS, but by short-term political advantage:

> *ML:* We have to resist the quick-fix mentality. There are two views of general management. The first is that it's something that you implement. The Department seems to have this view. I don't know what it is. Somehow you're supposed to implement it and then get back to the job. The other view is that it takes time, courage and that we will make mistakes. If you look at some of what's being done in the name of general management, it displays all the signs of the quick-fix mentality:

the disenfranchisement of nurses; the introduction of clinical budgeting without involving clinicians.

Pressured by immediate circumstance, or so it was argued, politicians con-stantly changed the rules under which the new managers were operating. One DGM noted the way this undermined his district's plans. Another ruefully compared her problems with ministers to her difficulties with clinicians:

*DGM:* The main thing I'm learning about in this job is politics. Once you're in the national network, there are all these major potential shifts in stance to deal with. The one that concerns me at the moment is the [government's change of mind on the] sale of residential accommodation – having built our capital plan around that! You build your plan and the sands shift under you.

*DGM:* Neither [doctors or nurses] take a wider view . . . Professional advice is fine about individual things but clinicians just can't take a global view. (*pause*) In fact, it's awfully difficult for any of us – that's why ministers keep on coming up with these initiatives which completely get in the way of their supposed national priorities!

Most crucially of all, managers believed that ministers and civil servants were flagrantly partial when they talked of decentralized decision making. Lower tiers might certainly be forced to devolve – but would the centre really give up all that accumulated power? Many senior managers in the early stages of Griffiths had their doubts:

*DCh:* It took them eleven months to appoint Victor Paige [the first chief executive of the NHS] . . . [The last time I was involved in a major business appointment] it took us a weekend! And if I'd been appointed I'd have insisted on a separate office that was seen to be separate from the minister – and from the civil service. Instead of which, he's been plonked in an office next to Kenneth Clarke [Minister for Health] and he writes letters off the same word-processor! . . . There's been some good appointments [to the NHS management board], of course. The finance director is a nice man. But it took him six months to discover that management budgeting would take time, instead of the ten days it would have taken him if he'd been allowed to get out and about. Instead, he was sent off on an induction course. Hopeless!

*DGM:* It's much tougher to change the Department than the NHS! . . . Griffiths is very good but it's not been very well implemented. It was wrong to appoint any general managers before the chief manager [Victor Paige] was appointed . . . Some-one told me that when Jim Phillips [a senior civil servant] was asked if he accepted Griffiths, he said 75 per cent. The 25 per cent he had doubts about was the centre! The bit that hasn't changed is the DHSS. The management board is just part of it. The DHSS needs no more than a hundred staff – it could do well with fifty – then it could deal with the strategic problems. As it is, well I got a frantic phone call last Thursday from the Minister's secretary, because he was being pressured by another minister over some little building we're selling to a local charity! You have to ask yourself, should the Secretary of State be responding to issues like that! . . . I don't think there's any broad strategic guidance from the centre. If the NHS management board disappeared tomorrow, no one would notice.

*DCh:* I was at a political dinner sitting next door to the Minister. We were intro-duced and he asked me was I enjoying it. I could have said, 'Yes. It is a great challenge'. But that would have been boring. So I said, 'Which do you want to hear, the standard reply or the truthful one?' He looked rather disconcerted and an aide stepped in and said, 'The truthful one'. So I said, 'I've been appointed as chairman and I don't mind giving or receiving orders. I don't mind at all. But having given us orders, would you please go away and let us get on with it. If you don't like what we do, sack us. But please let us get on with it. I run my own companies. They're pretty profitable. But I'm not allowed to run my health authority.' It's ridiculous that I have to get permission to appoint a DGM. Ludicrous. And in some districts they have changed the rules halfway through . . . There are interminable consultations above and below on almost any matter of consequence with region, the Minister, the borough, the staff consultative committees. And consultation is being confused with decision making. I might consult with you – but are we freely deciding together, or am I listening to you and then deciding? Too many organizations have a view that they have to input into the decision making.

## Who holds the purse-strings?

Another crucial deviation from the pure model of general management concerned funding and borrowing. In the new 1984 NHS, money was still allocated as it had been since 1948. It was top down, rather than bottom up. Instead of stemming from transactions with individual clients, finance came from the centre, trickling down to region, then to district, then to unit. As such, so some managers argued, the system removed an important element of consumer power. NHS patients lacked the choice available to others:

> DCh: Our customers are different from others. Few have the luxury of choice; few can complain because of the fear of retribution; few have the power to challenge the medical mystique.

> PSGM: [One of the] questions I get asked very, very frequently is, 'What does the private sector bring to health care?' . . . What my company does bring is a consumer-oriented aspect to even the smallest details of its work . . . Why do we give consultants primacy? Well, because patients choose us because of our consultants . . . Our customers are only there because they want to be . . . Success with our customers determines a private hospital's continued existence . . . Show me a patient who has had difficulty in getting a car-parking space and I'll show you a patient who's in need of tender loving care from the administration . . . We use questionnaires and follow-up phone interviews by nurses every month asking about suggestions for improved service.

The funding system had, so it was held, many other problematic consequences. One was that greater efficiency could mean more not less expense. In the following exchange at a management conference, the first speaker had developed a prize-winning system which had dramatically cut waiting lists and enabled many more patients to receive hip and knee replacements:

> DID: I should also say that it has cost us an extra quarter of a million pounds – mostly for spare parts for surgery . . .

*UGM:* In my district, we face a half million pound overspend this year. The last thing we want to see is more patients being treated! (*loud laughter*)

The absence of fee for service payment might not only penalize efficient individual services, it could also prevent them from raising their own money. This too might have serious effects on their efficiency; or so it was argued: .

*DFD:* Local authorities are funded in a much more sensible way – they can borrow and lend. In health authorities, however, we get simple cash allocations. I try and promote cost-consciousness, but in local authorities it's much sharper because you've got the cost of borrowing and the time of borrowing. But in health authorities, you go through all kinds of purely paper exercises. For example, if you're given money to construct a building the cost is related to the cost of capital on the money market. But because capital comes to us as a free gift on a non-recurring basis, therefore we tend not to be so cost-conscious.

The NHS system of central funding was also held to have disastrous effects on the quality of its management. That management might often have been weak – but just who was to blame? Though ministers talked of the vital need to contain the costs of NHS administration and insisted that the new structures be cheaper than the old, the new managers fundamentally disagreed. For all their enthusiasm for general management – and despite Drucker's thesis about the public sector's proneness to bureaucracy – there was a pervasive view that management was seriously under-funded and that this, in turn, had had seriously deleterious effects on the efficiency of the service as a whole. The politicians' desire to hold down public sector pay meant that the NHS had long had serious difficulties in attracting a cadre of first-class managers:

*DGM:* In my view, there's just not a sufficiently strong management structure at present. It is manageable, but we're very pushed to do it.

*DGM:* The NHS is under-managed certainly. And there's no money for new district management posts in the Griffiths reorganization, nor for getting staff for units. I think we're under-resourced for the scale of the task we're trying to tackle.

Below the most senior management posts, the pay was simply insufficient to attract competent staff:

*DCh:* As to personalities, at a higher level, they're very good . . . on a lower level, they're very often disappointing. The difficulty underneath district level is to find people competent to do the job . . . I think its the pay and the prospects for say the middle-ranking treasurer. In the finance department, there are just three people who can count on a five-figure salary. Everyone else is below that. Apart from the top job, it's not much of a wage.

*DGM:* In any competent industry, they'd have two or three accountants at unit level, but the NHS just can't afford that at the moment.

*DFD:* All this [financial devolution to units] means significant investment in accountants' time. If we under-invest, its credibility is lost. I recently summarized the immediate demands of the UGMs for accountants – we've got agreement on a new structure that supports the units and which will cost £25,000 more than previously.

Will this be enough? No – and we've said so . . . There's not much point in the government saying that NHS ought to adopt all these commercial approaches if they don't provide the facilities to enable this.

*UGM:* The man in charge of my outpatients department – which has a budget of five and a half million pounds – is paid just £11,500!

Finally, because health authorities were dependent on government allocations, while the volume of work bore no relation to their authorities' income, the entire health service had historically been funded on a largely external and often erratic basis. Indeed, it had often been at the mercy of the overall economy. When times were thought to be good, governments had been tempted to use the NHS as a means of expanding the general economy; vice versa when times were bad. Times were currently bad. In the 1980s, Griffiths was not the only force to shake the service as a whole. Of perhaps lesser importance, but attracting far greater publicity, was a major squeeze on most public sector expenditure. The squeeze had begun nearly a decade earlier and under a Labour not a Conservative government. Indeed, with the benefit of hindsight, many observers dated the onset of Thatcherism, not from 1979 when the Tories took office, but from that date three years earlier when the International Monetary Fund had imposed stringent conditions on government spending. The health service, for the first time, was held very strictly to its budgets. Districts which overspent now had to find the money from reserves or from next year's expenditure. As one minister said at the time, the party was over. The huge burst of growth in welfare expenditure which had begun in the 1960s had come to an end:

*CNA:* Up till 76, money wasn't an issue. If you spent more than you were allocated you got your fingers rapped, but you were still allocated more! . . . Then cash limits came in.

As a result, the districts we studied were obsessed, not just with Griffiths but with expenditure too:

*INT:* What are the most important things [for your DGM]?
*CNA:* Money!

Money was what health authority members spent most of their time discussing. Money was something that had been in short supply in the health service – with the brief exception of the 1960s – right from its very inception. Money was now, perhaps more than ever, the central topic on the agenda. After nearly a decade of cash limits, an acute financial crisis affected most units, districts and regions in the NHS, a crisis that had only been reinforced by the new government's emphasis on economy. 'Cost-improvement', as the drive was coyly known, bit deep. The pressure was intense:

*CNA:* He [UGM] is really going [he was resigning from his new post] because the job is impossible. They're the ones that are really being squeezed. He can't bear screwing people into the ground when they're already giving everything they've got . . . It's the UGMs in the acute services who are demoralized.

Overall expenditure still continued to rise, but the increase was far from sufficient to keep pace with the demands on the service. On every side there was mounting financial pressure: from the international exchanges, from the workforce, from new diseases, from new technological developments:

*DFD:* Where's Brian's nasty little point about oil stocks?
*DEO:* This is the point about cost-improvement on oil. When we come to do stock taking at the end of the year, the value of the oil in the tanks is £100,000 less than it was before . . . You've had the savings of the oil price fall. You've taken it off me to the tune of £230,000, I think, at the last count.

*DGM:* What do you make of the Chancellor's estimate of inflation?
*DFD:* I think he may be being optimistic.
*DGM:* Have you heard anything at all on nurses' pay yet?
*CNA:* No, but there's a lot of pressure to have special duties added in. I don't think that will be accepted, but I do think it will be more than 4.7 per cent.
*DFD:* Let's hope that it's not more than 5.7 per cent, otherwise we're in real trouble.

*DGM:* Our resources are deteriorating so rapidly . . . by next year, we're going to have to go for reductions in the service, not just holding things steady. And on top of this, of course, there is pressure for new services, for cervical screening and breast screening and hip replacement and AIDS. In AIDS the primary cases are going elsewhere, it's the long-term care that is going to be a problem here. We've had twenty cases so far and already had a 40-year-old dementing. The fudge over what you do about services like these is going to be harder and harder to achieve . . . the old-style British compromise of fudging between things is coming under great pressure . . . At the end of the day, it's a question of the sort of society we want. Having to make choices when provision is being reduced is extremely divisive . . . but that is the road we are being pushed towards. The potential for doing nothing for the old, the mentally ill and the socially useless is tremendous.

In some areas, the consequences were unclear. Did the current financial retrenchment stiffen resistance to the new general management – or actually force people to take a fresh look at old practices? Managers disagreed:

*RNO:* Any fool can manage when you're playing Father Christmas.

*DFD:* We've had some lovely examples of nurses who, when they saw cuts coming, have said, 'If we did X, Y, and Z, we'd save and avoid cuts'. Now it's the unit's money it's changed things.

However, although managers might disagree here, in one key matter the effects of such erratic funding seemed obvious. Compared with some other industrial countries, much of the capital stock was in urgent need of replacement, while far too many of the newer buildings were poorly built and maintained. Indeed, the last twenty-five years had seen an extraordinary cycle of boom and bust in NHS capital funding:

*DEO:* The NHS was a huge culture shock to me. I'd come from high-tech industry. Money was very easy. I came to the NHS where everything was run down and there was no professionalism at all on the estates side . . . The thing that attracted me in was Powell's [1962] hospital building plan. To rebuild all the hospitals they needed professional leadership. Someone qualified like me was rare. Most of the guys on the works side were upgraded plumbers or electricians . . . The hospital management committee was a farce . . . It was all run on the back of an envelope . . . It never spent any money except on day to day things . . . I remember one meeting, one of the surgeons was deputed to go and sort out the boiler-house! They wrote a letter to region saying they should switch to mains electricity! Everything in the hospital was on non-standard voltage . . . The Tyler Report on hospital engineering came out in 1965 and ushered in a huge period of change. I was caught up very quickly in rebuilding. I was appointed to sort out the maintenance but there was no time for that. My first job was to sort out the Part Three accommodation at the old work-house. The hospital secretary was formerly the workhouse master. It had two floors, one male and one female. I can picture it now. Old ladies huddling round a fire in a Nightingale ward! It was positively Dickensian . . . I had to convert these into single-bedded accommodation for nurses – all of them recruited from abroad, mainly the West Indies. They were living in even worse accommodation in what had been a home for tramps and hadn't changed much since . . . New contracts appeared almost every other week. We were spending money like water. And the faster you spent the money, the more resources you got! We never closed anything down, we always expanded . . . They set up the 74 reorganization to cope with all this. And having got a good system to cope with expansion – and plan for more – straightaway in 74 we found ourselves having to contract. And it's been more so ever since. To the point where we are going to fall apart unless we get some more cash . . . We've just surveyed all the buildings and we need £12.2 million just to put the backlog of maintenance right! Everywhere you touch in the NHS has got financial problems. Everywhere it's a scandal.

## Devolution from region?

The new general management was therefore still trapped inside the old NHS hierarchy, with its political interference and its central allocation of funding. Indeed, central control affected every tier of the organization. If Whitehall often refused to devolve so, in their turn, did the regions, as they gazed fearfully up to their political masters – or so some district managers argued:

*CNA:* The RGM and RCh have toed the political line from above. There are lots of jokes that Charles Adams [RCh] would do anything for a knighthood!

*DCh:* I am constantly frustrated about the very confused and ill-thought out lines of communication between us and region and the Department. You either make it a proper corporate structure or you get rid of regions.

*DFD:* The Minister is going up the wall apparently about the way the figures have been presented, the way they suggest there's been a net reduction in resources – he argues that it's due to the effect of the pay award . . . He's now blaming the region which is hard luck on them. It's not their fault . . . I feel sorry for them.
*DGM:* Don't feel at all sorry. They've fudged it.

*CNA:* They put out that press release.

*DFD:* Yes, that was unforgivable.

*DGM:* There was a complete lack of discussion with the districts. And when we tried to raise it with them, they just lost their temper. There was no advance warning at all of a complete change in line. In these days of general management, they should use the network and inform the DGM or the chairman.

Thus, some district managers felt that instead of paying attention to what was happening on the ground, their region persisted with top down and unrealistic plans through obeying the political and civil service tiers. Despite the general management philosophy, the centre still thought that it alone knew best. In the following extract, for example, district managers discussed their current staffing and the way this conflicted with regional plans:

*DPO:* Basically, what the table on page 5 shows is what's happening to manpower. What it shows is that we're moving in the opposite direction to what's planned . . . So I've written a new strategy based on our present needs.

*DGM:* How is region taking this?

*CNA:* Maureen [RNO] is very unhappy about us saying anything other than that we're trying to achieve the plan.

*DPO:* I had a regional document last week saying that they were still hoping to meet the target figures at the end of the decade.

*DGM:* This is absolutely lunatic. I said to them last week that it was absolutely lunatic and they should abandon it. Bertrand [RCh] said I was being outrageous and defeatist – and that the plan would *have* to be implemented; ha! ha! [Original emphasis]

*CNA:* Maureen [RNO] said that region intends to carry out the plan and that unless we put bids in we won't get anything.

*DGM:* I think it's better not to go along with region, get told off, and then expose what they've said.

*DFD:* I agree. I think there's a lot to be said for planning realistically.

The managers of this district were particularly outspoken but there were similar complaints from those in districts which took a less independent line:

*DGM:* One of my biggest worries about region is that there's no one at the top who has had any experience of working at an operational level since 1974 and yet the service has changed out of all recognition – and it shows.

*DGM:* [This is a very big region] there is no single individual that I can ring up and they'd say, 'Oh, it's so-and-so, we know about it, this is what's happening'. So in fact it gets very frustrating.

Finally, consider the way in which regions could regularly offend districts over regional specialisms – services for the rarer conditions which were based in just one hospital in a region and treated patients from all the surrounding local districts. The district in whose hospital such a service was based could face major problems over its control. Some regions, so it was argued, treated these services as entirely their own, even though developments within them had major implications for local staffing and finance. Consider this extract from a district management meeting:

> *DGM:* This is a fascinating letter [promising regional money for medical develop-ments in a specialism based in the district]. I thought I'd just show it to you . . . Apparently Philip [RGM] met Steven [a consultant at the district DGH] at some do and told him he'd be able to get money for new developments in his [medical] unit. And this was exactly at the same time as we heard from region about their plans and there was no mention of any developments in this unit at all! It was absolutely at the bottom of their priorities. He's just a boy who can't say no!
>
> *DFD:* This last paragraph is meaningless. No one in that [medical] unit has ever been able to control workload.
>
> *CNA:* My fear at the moment is that it's an open-ended commitment. For eight years, The Princess [DGH] has been taking money from the rest of the service in order to fund it.
>
> *DGM:* I quite agree with you. District is subsidizing these people. Region recog-nizes this but does nothing about it.
>
> *CNA:* And it's not recognized in the nursing budget.

## Devolution from district?

But, of course, if districts complained about region and Whitehall, units in their turn complained about district. Every superior tier had the potential to oppress the inferior layers. Loud shouts about the sins of those above might merely drown out the screams from those below. As we saw earlier, very large districts with a big population and many different hospitals could face major problems in reducing their number of units. To go for just a few units might mean that each was unwieldy, to go for many could mean an over-large district management board. Of course, where the UGMs were excluded from the board, the district officers still stressed that they were careful to consider the interests of each unit:

> *CNA:* We're very careful at district level to avoid any discussions about the oper-ational groups [units] – and they [UGMs] do come along [to board meetings] from time to time if there are key issues.

However, the rationale given by district could be seen rather differently from the perspective of unit. Were the old officers simply conspiring against the new general management?

> *UGM:* This district's got very peculiar UGM arrangements. The UGMs are not participating nearly as much in the decision making as they ought to be. There's too much strength in the executive board – which we're not on . . . I'm not the only one to think this . . . Shirley [DGM] probably felt that the old DMT was working well and she'd got the existing officers behind her – so there was no point in rocking the boat and changing the structure . . . The issue of the UGMs being on the board has never been raised . . . I expect the UGMs who were administrators feel it less because their role hasn't changed so much. If the board wasn't as strong, the role of some of the officers, for example X and Y [the professional advisors] would be much less influential than it is now.

This UGM was based in a very large district, whose problems might well seem a special case. But, whatever a district's size, structure, history and capital stock, there was always, so it seemed, plenty of room for continuing tension between districts and units. The new district management was very keen to assert its overall authority. The following quotations come from three much smaller districts:

> *CNA:* One of the difficulties at district is poor communication. We are still having role conflict between the UGMs and the chief officer group. We met separately with the UGMs but that was stopped before Christmas and now we meet together – but there is still suspicion.

> *DGM:* He [UGM] began to identify solely with the unit and to think that there was no need for the district level . . . He was at loggerheads with all my directors.

> *DMO:* Lots of district administrators who became UGMs thought they'd do everything, that they'd be in charge. But in fact it's the DGM. So it's a culture shock. The unit administrator used to be the bee's knees. They had much more power relative to the district administrator than the UGM has in relation to the DGM. So it's been a real shock!

> *DGM:* The units in this district were almost completely autonomous. That had been the previous policy. When I came, I found a lot of playing off of unit against district and unit against unit. There was no overall identification as a district. The DNSs paid no respect to the DNO. There was no acknowledgement of her existence. So at my first authority meeting, I pointed out that the acute unit wasn't actually making efficiency savings. Instead, it was just top-slicing money off the nursing budget in order to balance the unit budget. So I took some financial control back to district . . . It was fascinating coming from X district . . . There, there were district plans which we tried to get the units identifying with. Here they were totally separate and very aggressive towards each other.

The government, then, had introduced a modern business model of organization but had done so inside the traditional health service hierarchy. Frontline managers were now supposed to innovate but they could only do this within tight bureaucratic controls and under major central constraints over funding. The new devolution was not all that ministers claimed it to be. But the problems of hierarchy did not stop there. In the final part of this chapter, we consider two more crucial problems with money and power that the national model made for the new general managers. A national health service had meant, not just a national management hierarchy, but a national system of both punishment and pay. As a result, local managers often lacked both the capacity to reward loyal service and the power to sanction that of which they disapproved.

### The power to reward?

At the core of general management doctrine was a focus on performance. Where NHS staff had once been accountable solely to their tribe, Griffiths had set out to break down the old divisions. Every doctor, nurse, manager, porter was now to be both part of a corporate team and simultaneously a lone individual whose contribution to that team was routinely monitored and assessed. A new team with a new method of organization required a new sort of motivation. Professional ethics and aspirations were to be matched – or replaced – by a new stress on individual incentives. But, in practice, the new NHS was powerfully shaped by the old ways. Pay was still determined, not by local managers' assessment of worth and of need, but by national agreements with professions and unions. District might vary from district in a thousand and one ways but their pay scales were uniform and inflexible:

> DGM: Last year I stayed with some friends in the States who run hospitals. We talked about pay bargaining. If I want to get a salary variation for a member of staff I have to go to the DHSS and it's all done in the name of a member of the Cabinet! They couldn't believe it. I believe very strongly in local pay bargaining. We need to reward individual merit. I believe we [DGMs] should get an allocation and how we allocate it is up to us – though the principles could be based on open debate. But we're completely debarred from doing this.

Such inflexibility applied to many levels:

> DGM: How are we going to get ward sisters into general management if, in fact, her boss earns less than she does?

> RFD: Why haven't consultants been involved in Griffiths more?
> UGM (ex-doctor): Unless we put our money where our mouth is, consultants won't do any more outside their own area.

> CNA: We're desperately hoping that Whitley will come up with as loose a system for clinical nurses as it has for managers. I want to break the salary system down from the present inflexible system to a merit or results system.

Indeed, so powerful were the traditional, national methods for setting pay and rewards that even the new management suffered from exactly the same problem. It, at least, was supposed to be flexible (as the last speaker indicated) but there were still bizarre variations in the terms offered to managers from different backgrounds and some extraordinarily lengthy delays in fixing payments for additional responsibilities:

> DGM: My first UGM came in January and my acute UGM in March. Their salaries still aren't fixed. It's daft. There's been an abysmal hiatus. There's been very great uncertainty; it's very debilitating for everyone. It's gone on since June . . . The Department [DHSS] has been changing its mind every five minutes.

> DGM: I was conscious I was taking a gamble as it's a short-term contract and, as a nurse, I lost my conditions of service – whereas doctors [who go into general management] are protected. And you couldn't negotiate on salaries. Frankly, I'm not getting a lot more than I did as a DNO – just a couple of thousand more.

> DCh: It's all Yes, Minister to a degree – we've got an NHS management board who do nothing except write letters about cockroaches! Poor Jim [DGM who is also a doctor] still only gets £2,750 on top of his medical salary . . .
> . . . INT: [The same district fifteen months later] What's your own future as a general manager?

*DGM:* Ha! Ha! I'm more than two years through my three-year contract and they still haven't given me a contract!

*DNE/CNA:* I generally leave home at 7 am, am here from about 7.45 and I usually get home about 8 pm.
*INT:* You are still on a DNE's salary.
*DNE/CNA:* Yes, a grade 3. It has absolutely not changed since I took this on. Initially [fifteen months previously] I said to my wife, 'Don't worry . . . some extra payment will come' – and that hasn't happened. I am supposed to be getting a variation order from the DHSS; an allowance will be given . . . It's still waiting at the DHSS . . . I can't reassure her that this is coming and that her loss of my time was worthwhile . . . Two of the [DNSs] are more senior than I am in terms of salary . . . We used to have a DNO that got about £27,000 or £30,000 year – there's their savings.

## The power to discipline?

If pay was still inflexible and devolution not all it was cracked up to be, the most crucial compromise of all concerned discipline. Griffiths was all about letting managers manage. Yet the 1984 reorganization had failed to face up to medical syndicalism. The might of the nationally organized medical workforce meant that the new local leaders were still unable to manage the dominant clinical trade. Though the new reforms drew heavily on American inspiration, DGMs and UGMs lacked the fundamental power available to American hospital managers. American managers had the ability to discipline or even remove those doctors who did not step into line. But in Britain, although the government had taken on the miners, the doctors – thus far – remained untouched:

*CNA:* Griffiths was asking for far more skilled managers than he realized because he was really asking for managers who could manage without having sanctions over doctors.

*DFD:* We need medical chiefs of service, like they've got in the USA [where each medical service had a medical manager]. We can't really continue to deal with individual consultants. But whether at Guy's they'll be able to carry the day, I don't know. [Guy's Hospital in London was attempting to apply the American system.] The key is can we [DFD mimes cutting their throats]? The ideal solution is to have chiefs of staff who have real power – then you're cooking with gas. But in the absence of that, it's a bumpy road.

*DGM:* There are ways to control doctors but they are not available to us yet and they won't be for five years or more.

Moreover, not only did doctors continue to have exceptional powers, but there was some organized professional resistance to any external monitoring of medical performance:

*UGM:* In North America and Australia, doctors are much more prepared to accept that they have a corporate and not just an individual responsibility for the quality of care. I've had a real debate with the local medical committee over this. The BMA has not done us any great service. Their evidence to the Royal Commission in 1977 stated, 'We are not convinced of the need for further supervision of a qualified doctor's standard of care'. The United States has got a much better system of post-qualification supervision . . . In the USA the onus is increasingly on the doctor to prove that they can stay; but in the UK the onus is on the authority to try and get rid of them.

The matter of sanctions was, however, a delicate affair. Though the outside world may associate general management with tough action, general managers themselves, at least publicly, rarely touched on the power to sack. A leading businessman and prophet of general management, who addressed health service managers on the new methods, laid great stress on the fundamental nature of teamwork and the crucial importance of incentives but, strikingly, made no mention of his power to discipline. Likewise, even the American managers from Johns Hopkins Medical School – here to show the NHS just how it could be done – emphasized the necessity of winning medical consent but made no allusion whatsoever (at least in their formal presentations) to their formidable power to sanction recalcitrant doctors. Such revelations were left to question time:

> *HSR:* In your talk on clinical budgeting, you haven't mentioned the power that you have over your doctors.
> *USGM:* . . . All our doctors are on two-year contracts – but we give them a year's notice if we want to get rid of them . . . The chief of service [a doctor] carries a lot more clout than anyone comparable in the NHS. The chief is appointed by the Dean and the Director . . . There's been a big change of heart in the last five years. Most of the chiefs of service are now very management oriented and very rational – they're data oriented. If a physician's length of stay is way out of line
> *RFD:* You break their thumbs!
> *USGM:* – He'll be seen by the director of the unit; if it's still out, he gets a phone call from me – and even from the [hospital] president himself. A lot of the old chiefs left. They didn't like the management style. The new ones do and work well inside it.

In Britain, however, given doctors' lifetime contracts and the power of medical syndicalism, it was almost impossible for managers to remove them. It could just be done, but even in the most damning of circumstances, took many years of struggle and extraordinary effort:

> *CNA:* [Parking his car in a space labelled 'Dr Maclean'] I always park here! Dr Maclean has been suspended for two years. It was a dreadful case. If it had been a nurse she'd have gone immediately. Doctors' cases can drag on for at least five years, what with appeals and so on.

> *DGM:* We've just sacked a consultant. It was discussed in the private session [of the health authority meeting]. He was absolutely hopeless – taking drugs, high all the time, giving the wrong treatments, falling off chairs in meetings and so on. He was reported to the GMC who suspended him – but eventually they wanted him returned to an ordinary physician's job. The RMO went along with this [consultants' contracts were held at region, not at district] but I went to him and said, 'Look, I want him out'. The RMO thought I'd gone mad but he backed me in the end. It was a huge battle. It was discussed by the RHA and I insisted that the DHA

members saw the transcripts of the evidence that had been sent to the RHA. It wasn't seen as any of their business, but I insisted. They were absolutely shocked – particularly by the evidence that if junior doctors had followed the consultant's instructions people might have died. The appeal went all the way to the Secretary of State. If it hadn't gone our way, I'm certain that one of our members would have leaked the documents to the press and then there'd have been a huge public stink!

Sacking doctors demanded extraordinary sins and equally extraordinary time and effort from everyone else concerned. It was, therefore, useless as an every day management sanction. Moreover, not only did doctors have the power to resist many features of general management, they might even have the power to shape just who got appointed as a manager in the first place. Ministers might urge that nurses come forward to enter general management but some who had done so spoke of the severe resistance they had encountered, as a nurse, from the medical profession:

> *DGM:* I applied to X [the district where she had previously been DNO] but the doctors wouldn't permit someone like me getting a job . . . Then I could have got Y district but the doctors there overruled it. There was resistance here too but it wasn't as strong – though everyone told me in my first month that many of the doctors didn't want me.

Finally, by contrast, consider managers' power to discipline nurses. Unlike doctors, they were readily dismissed for taking drugs or maltreating patients; indeed such discipline was a major preoccupation for nurse managers and the threat of dismissal hung, like Damocles' sword, over clinical nursing practice. Removing nurses for other reasons was, however, quite a different matter. Nurses too had considerable security in their conditions of employment. Though far less of a challenge to the new general management, this still constrained the full application of the business model:

> *RCN representative:* Nurses can be made redundant or they can be found alternative employment. There's a lot of scope for that in the NHS . . . [But] I can count the cases of redundancies that I've ever heard of on the fingers of one hand . . . Nurses do enjoy a greater degree of tenure than most other people in the public sector, let alone elsewhere.

## Conclusion

Griffiths, then, for all its radicalism, was only a partial break with the past. There was now a chain of command which reached from the top to the bottom of the organization. There was also a new headquarters staff with a potential flexibility to match the exigencies of local need and form. But the service was still trapped, for general managers at least, within a national straitjacket. Local initiative was frustrated by ministers, by civil servants, by supervisory management tiers and by powerful professional bodies. Doctors still gave orders, nanny still knew best.

# 11      Efficiency and effectivenes

The first chapter in this assessment of Griffiths stressed the way in which it compromised with the past. The 1984 reorganization was a mixture of modern business management with the very different traditions of national and professional monopoly. Many managers felt that the compromise was an awkward one. Still, Griffiths was only a beginning, a first step down a long road. Politicians might learn not to interfere; civil servants, regions and districts might learn to devolve; managers might be given fresh powers to deal at long last with clinical medical power.

There was, however, one other fundamental problem with Griffiths; a problem which might prove even more difficult to solve. For general management was a doctrine, not just of firm leadership and corporate structure, but of cost and quality too. General management was only a new means to the old end of better organizational performance. But better results could be guaranteed only if the new managers knew what they were doing. The new leaders needed more powers than they had had in the past but, just as crucially, they needed better information if performance was now to be measured and improved. How was this to be done?

This chapter explores the many profound difficulties which beset the attempts to develop better NHS information. It reviews the fierce debates over the quality and implementation of the new information systems, the doubts as to whether the new measures actually measured performance, the strange absence of basic research into many fundamental management issues, and the continuing vexed problems over professional advice. Above all, however, it considers the potentially major contradictions between the two key goals of the new general management. Griffiths was a determined assault on two fronts: on cost and on quality. Yet, as Drucker had warned general managers, whatever they did, they must not substitute the first for the second. Consider his arguments once again:

> Service institutions need people who do the management job systematically and who focus themselves and their institution purposefully on performance and results. They do need efficiency – that is, control of costs – but above all they need effectiveness – emphasis on the right results.[1]

Yet here too, as we shall now see, some of the new managers had apparently forgotten or ignored the doctrine in whose name they ruled. Too often, or so it seemed to some of their colleagues, some new general managers resembled the old clinical managers they had overthrown. If DMOs and DNOs had been massively parochial, many DGMs and UGMs, DFDs and UFDs might well be just the same. Most had the best of motives but, knowing little or nothing of the product itself, they were forced to concentrate on its cost. Trapped once again within their own disciplines – this time of administration and accountancy – they focused solely on efficiency and bothered little, if at all, about quality – or so sceptics argued. Quality might be a shining new goal, an ever-present slogan, the catchphrase of the moment. But if one examined what most managers did, not just what they mouthed, only some seemed to take quality seriously. Others, so it appeared, just did not know what it actually meant. All kinds of naive notions abounded, from the very top to the bottom of the management tree. To many observers, cost, cost and then cost again was what really counted. It was the only thing most politicians or managers knew much about, the only thing that could readily be quantified. Of course, there were exceptions, but in far too many places, the old incompetence had merely been replaced by the new ignorance – or so some feared.

## The right information?

For general management to work according to the model, there must not only be devolution and the proper mix of sanctions and incentives, but relevant, precise and up-to-date information. One manager put the problem like this:

> *DGM:* What I can't answer is, 'Is Mrs Jones in the second bed from the left getting the same quality of treatment that she was two years ago?' I can't answer that – and I need to know.

Such information was an absolute necessity for every level of the organization. But, for all the great stress on information and the many attempts to introduce new types of information system, there were serious difficulties. One important worry, so both British and American managers argued, was the way data could be rejected, reinterpreted or even falsified:

> *RGM:* If PIs [performance indicators] are seen as the studs in the jackboot, all kinds of games will be played. People will just reject the accuracy of the information.

> *USGM:* People are brilliant at beating the system. There's a lot of clever people in medical centres and all of them are obsessive compulsives! So, if there's a very dramatic change in the figures you have to be suspicious. We say to them, you can make a mistake once (*pause*) but if it happens again (*pause*) they'd better have some very good evidence of what's been going on to justify it.

Moreover, not only might data be mistrusted or misused, but in many key areas the data that existed were hardly usable. Past inadequacies and severe technical problems beset almost every information system:

*RGM (at management conference):* Does anyone here know the proportion of cancelled operations in their hospital?
*Audience:* Yes, Yes, Yes.
*RGM:* I don't believe you. I don't believe you.

*CNA:* Quality assessment won't work until we've got the right data sets. The NHS is full of rubbishy information that we don't need.

*DFD:* Changes in technology have facilitated far more active financial management. It may have gone too far. Because the technology is there, the demands for ever more action grow. But whether managers are able to use all this information is debatable. Well, not debatable – they *can't* use it on a routine basis. The next step, though we're not there yet, is to provide information on demand rather than *en masse* – when it's overwhelming. [Original emphasis]

There was, therefore, far too much useless or inaccurate information and, at the same time, far too little serious information on many crucial points:

*Surgeon:* I'm here [at this conference] with my theatre manager – who'll no doubt refute everything I say! As a doctor, I'm a bit dubious about statistics. For example, you [speaker] were worried about the variation in the length of time spent in pre-op. Well, it all depends, for example, on whether there's a new SHO [senior house officer], and on training time – and that sort of information is missing [from the system you describe]. You asked in your last question was there too much information or too little. I'd say too little.

All this was worrying enough. What led to even more concern was the fear that very few serious steps were being taken to remedy the situation. As we have seen, a key instruction from Whitehall during the implementation of Griffiths had been that there should be no overall increase in management costs. Yet, while the NHS was sometimes held to be absurdly bureaucratic, its administrative costs were, in fact, extraordinarily low compared with the businesses on which it now had to model itself. Even more worryingly, while such businesses spent far more on their information systems, their information needs were much less complex than those of the NHS:

*MC:* How much is this going to cost? [The new attempt to assess the costs of individual treatment.] All this is going to be very expensive . . .

*DFD:* The Department has considerably underestimated the expense in my view. I think there's a funny notion going around that we can get by with a fairly modest amount and just small data-capture systems. The potential for savings is large but the costs can be very large – and education and training to use the systems can also be very expensive.

*CNA:* It has to be remembered [in the debate over developing quality] that Sainsbury's management costs are 13 per cent [i.e. roughly three times higher than the formal management costs of the NHS – Roy Griffiths had come to the NHS from the supermarket chain, Sainsbury's] . . .

*HSR:* That's a very relevant point. Quantifiable measures of quality can be developed but it will cost big money – several per cent of the NHS budget.

Not only were there serious doubts about the level of investment, but the speed at which the national, regional and district tiers introduced the new systems was also of fundamental concern. Both politicians and general managers were faced with the threat of re-election or reappointment. Had things, therefore, been done far too fast?

> *MC:* What worries me is the practical implementation of all these things. It all looks very nice but the pace at which people are instructed to implement things in X region is absurd. For example, districts have been told to implement Korner [a new routine NHS information system] before the new computer systems have been introduced. So they're implementing Korner manually! I'm worried that if things are implemented quickly, they'll be done badly.
>
> *RFD:* I don't know how you can implement Korner manually!
>
> *HSR:* At the moment, people are rushed off their feet introducing all these different systems – and usually it's the same person having to do it. It's ridiculous.
>
> *UNO:* I don't think anyone listens. And if you dare raise your voice or question them then you're in trouble, because they want Monitor [a new nursing quality control system] . . . They say they want to put the district on the map. I have grave reservations about who it is they want to put on the map! I think over the past two or three years we have rushed into things headlong. If you rush those things, that are not properly thought through, not properly resourced, then for ground level staff that just leads to frustration.

One standard subject for such criticisms were the pilot management budgeting schemes (also known variously as clinical budgeting and resource management). Given its emphasis on macro- not micro-management, the old NHS had never calculated the cost of individual treatment. But, if doctors were to monitor their own expenditure and if the performance of one doctor was to be compared with another, a new costing methodology was essential. In several districts around the country, experimental systems had therefore been set up. Given the huge variety of medical conditions and medical treatment, such schemes were enormously complex. Moreover, it was generally agreed that they had been introduced at too fast a pace and without adequate training, consultation or resources:

> *MC:* X district was hopeless. They completely failed to educate the consultants. Those in charge of introducing the scheme to the district were so wrapped up in it that they didn't bother to explain it to anyone, while the consultants didn't dare ask. In my opinion, the Department brought the whole thing on far too fast. They should have experimented in just three or four favourable departments – not whole districts – and the time-scale should have been longer. Mind, it was all dreamed up by an accountant from a biscuit factory! Some people had warned against going too fast – I did – but ministers had insisted.

Speaking at a conference of finance directors, a member of the NHS management board confessed that there had been many grave difficulties:

> *NHSBM:* Two fundamental lessons can be drawn. One is that it's very much easier to develop and implement mechanical processes for disaggregating costs down to clinicians than it is to win the support of clinicians for the management budgeting

process. The second is that we have significantly under-estimated the financial and management resources needed to educate doctors to understand how it will help them with their problems . . . [Also] costing reports have mostly been indiscriminate. They've produced an awful lot of data on matters which doctors don't control or influence. The systems have been under-designed. More worryingly, even in the successful sites, the resources in the management and financial areas have been too small to respond to consultants' reasonable enquiries about the meaning of individual items of data.

To many, such observations seemed a little late in the day. Whitehall might have looked to America for inspiration, but it had clearly not looked very hard. Precisely these lessons were already available from the American pioneers of clinical budgeting. The managers at Johns Hopkins in Baltimore reported to the same conference just how they had done things. Unlike their British counterparts, they had taken things slowly and gone to great lengths to win the support of their clinicians – as the following exchange revealed:

*DFD:* We were under pressure to get the whole thing going in six months, yet you've been talking about two years!
*USGM:* Early on, we had masses of complaints about bad information. The data purification stage took two years. You can't have consultants walk away and say, 'This will never do!'

There were, then, fundamental problems with clinical budgeting. But this was not the only information system where such difficulties existed. The next two sections consider a pair of equally vital areas for the Griffiths reforms: the performance indicators created for each tier of management and the systems being developed to monitor the single largest item of NHS expenditure – nursing.

## Indicators of performance?

Clinical budgeting focused on the work of individual doctors. Since the NHS had never before collected such information, this was a most ambitious scheme; central to the future management of the NHS but still at an experimental stage. Another sort of performance indicator had, however, been created straight away by the new general management; one that relied, not on experimental but on traditional NHS information. It had long been possible, at least in principle, to compare the activity that took place in different regions and districts: how much was spent on this, how many patients were treated for that. But, while such information had been available before, it had never been used in any systematic fashion. Now, however, it became central to the work of the new centralized management and the chain of command that stretched from Whitehall to the ward. Comparative measures were created for each management tier, enabling those above to compare the aggregated activity that took place in the tiers below. The NHS management board could now monitor the regions, the regions could monitor the districts.

Yet, though these aggregated indicators were far simpler than clinical budgeting, they too had a very mixed reception. At best, they were viewed as of some use – but as only a beginning. At worst, they were seen as positively misleading. Managers were divided. For the enthusiasts, some comparison was better than none at all. Now, at long last, systematic questions could be asked about relative performance. For the sceptics, the questions were often pointless. If the old data sets were full of rubbish, why should questions based upon them be taken seriously? Moreover, were the right sorts of things being quantified? Even supposing some of the measures were accurate, did these new performance indicators actually measure performance? Perhaps the huge review system based upon them was largely wasted? Might it, indeed, seriously distort the running of the entire NHS? Opinions differed. Managers often swithered between one view and the other:

> *UGM:* I agree they don't provide much information. But these figures do at least enable us to start asking questions based on objective data. This is a beginning.

> *DGM:* The PI package will help a bit – but the basic thing is to build up local information which we can use with the consultants.

> *CNA:* Performance indicators can't stand alone. They're just like RAWP. They're very insensitive. I met a man from X district who thought that if there was an outlier, you needed to do something right away!

> *DGM:* I'm not going to be talking about PIs – the ones we have are not very good at the moment.

> *CNA:* I think national PIs are a pretty sterile exercise, they're mostly just inputs.

This last point refers to a key part of the critique. For some managers, performance indicators were a sign of a fundamentally misdirected national strategy; of an emphasis solely on inputs rather than outputs. The standard NHS information systems could measure, if often very crudely, just what went into health care: the numbers of staff, patients, or beds, and just what was spent at an aggregate level. What they could not do was assess the outcome of all this; how far patients' health actually improved as a result of such expenditure of time, money and resources. One district might well spend far more than another on paediatrics – perhaps, as a result, their children were far healthier. No one knew.

The difficulties in finding out were technically formidable. Formal health care, as most researchers argue, is just one ingredient in the generation of health; very often, perhaps, of far less account than genetics, tobacco, diet, housing, class or culture. Since districts varied so fundamentally in their size, wealth and population, variations in the health of their citizens were hardly surprising. Separating out the effects of one factor from another was a task that was still in its infancy. Moreover, health care itself was often an unknown quantity. Remarkably little was scientifically established about the effectiveness of many medical and nursing treatments. New, evaluative methodologies had been developed over the past few decades, but an enormous amount of costly and complex work remained to be done. Indeed, the task was never ending.

New treatments were constantly being developed and applied well before anyone knew much about their real worth.

None the less, for all these difficulties, only outcome measures could determine whether the NHS was getting serious quality, real value for money; or so researchers – and some managers – insisted. Here, then, was where information was most vitally needed. Detailed costing of health care was fine – but what use was knowledge of its cost, if basic information on its effectiveness was lacking? To these sceptics, the central place of PIs in NHS management review was symptomatic of a narrow and ignorant emphasis on immediate financial information:

> *RGM:* The management board has no idea about effectiveness. All they're interested in is efficiency.

Others argued, however, that these were merely academic doubts. PIs existed, outcome measures did not and action was needed now. Cost was crucial no less than quality and cost could be measured. Who knew how long the NHS would have to wait before there were serious measures of effectiveness?

Such differences in analysis and interest – and the major tensions these could produce – are clearly brought out in the following debate from another management conference. Here too, the day had begun with a speech from a member of the NHS management board; a speech which was brisk and bullish:

> *NHSBM:* There is now huge interest in NHS information. Measurement is very fashionable . . . Some managers may ask why the board is interested in measurement when at region and district the real battle is going on with shot and shell and there's no time at all for these fancy academic interests. But this is to mistake the skirmish for the real battle. There are too many important things going on at the moment to be into frippery. Nor, may I say, are we into it so that some obscure research institute in a downtown polytechnic can produce a few obscure PhDs which no one will ever read (*laughter*) . . . We are concerned with measurement to make ourselves more efficient. Over the last five years we have steadily increased productivity in terms of the numbers of patients being treated in relation to the numbers of staff and the amount of investment. But the continued wide range of variation [in health service activity levels] poses a number of questions. We've standardized many of the inputs so people can't plead special factors. What we have to do is to lift everyone from the bottom quartile to the mid-point. For the first time, the PI package offers us a major diagnostic tool. PIs also enable us to target our enormous resources onto patients. We need to be exact about what we're doing; for example, for particular age groups, or for prevention . . . And – somewhere over the horizon – we need to develop measures of outcome . . . Measurement of our activity is fundamental to progress. Without it we cannot give this great national service the impetus it deserves . . . Measurement, castigated by Burke as the tool of economists, calculators and sophists, has come out of the closet. We have an exciting time ahead of us!
>
> . . . *DGM:* Given that outcome is, as you say, over the horizon, will measurement techniques be applicable to outcome?
>
> *NHSBM:* I know the problem is enormously difficult. How it will be resolved and whether it will be resolved and whether we will like the results when we get them, I

do not know. However, I do know that developing measures of what we actually do is a necessary first step towards outcome measures – if that's what we want to do. It may turn out to be like the philosopher's stone.

By contrast, a health service researcher who spoke later in the morning was highly critical of the strategy as laid down by Whitehall:

*HSR:* Coming out of the closet, I am an economist and an academic! When I was asked to speak at this conference, I was also asked if I believed in PIs – and I said I was an agnostic. There's a lot of heat and dust, but I'm not sure. PIs are only a means to an end . . . Yet their introduction has preceded any serious discussion of objectives. The problem of objectives is however normally overwhelmed by the problem of measurement. What are we measuring? It is recognized that these are all throughput not outcome measures and they often depend on factors outside the health service, e.g. the social services. We also have to be concerned with particular types of efficiency. 'Economic efficiency' is concerned with the maximization of output from given levels of input . . . PIs extend purely financial monitoring by looking at the volume of throughput. They complement cash limits and their fundamental, though not exclusive, concern is cost-containment. Now, should cost-containment be our main concern? By international comparisons we spend very little and yet the nation's health is not noticeably worse off. So we're coping quite well. However, most health economists would argue we're not doing well with another type of efficiency – allocative efficiency – i.e. could we benefit more from allocating resources differently, for example, by giving less to geriatrics and more to acute services – or vice versa? This type of efficiency depends on having measures of outcome and the existing PIs fall a long way short of this. Some community physicians have been pushing for more work on effectiveness – but with not much success. Why has so little work been done here? Most NHS information is not addressed to issues of effectiveness. Instead, most of it is addressed to financial review, especially yearly review – which has led to incremental budgeting rather than trying to implement substantial changes in the overall mix of what we're doing. The best person to evaluate effectiveness, the clinician, often does not find it opportune to do so. We need to experiment more – but this of course is expensive. I find it slightly surprising that so many public resources are devoted to a service so much of which has not been shown to be effective.

The subsequent debate from the floor brought out strongly the contrast between the immediate needs that some general managers stressed and the doubts raised by most academics and some other managers about the utility of much that was currently being attempted:

*DCh:* I'm a convert to PIs. The question I want to ask the last speaker is what would he do if he were actually running the service rather than attending to academic interests. Looking at the variations, I'm struck by some extraordinary facts, e.g. that neonatal mortality varies by a factor of 10 and day surgery by a factor of 50.
*HSR1:* I'm not objecting to the direction the service is moving in. I just think we must be careful not to tread too narrow a path.
*DGM1:* . . . I think both sides are correct. What I want to know is, can the academics specify how much variation is acceptable? Fivefold is disgraceful, fiftyfold is a joke.

*HSR1:* You're right. The ones that are really hanging off the wall can be picked off easily – but what about the rest? How do we make sense of them?

*DGM2:* Isn't there a conflict between the culture of the academic – careful, rational, wanting all the information in to make rational decisions – and, on the other hand, that of the general manager – who's portrayed as a J. R. Ewing type? [A character in the soap opera *Dallas*] Can it be resolved?

*HSR1:* I don't know.

*HSR2:* I'm another one of those unsavoury academics! I want to turn the question back on the first questioner. Take, for example, a very high-cost prescribing GP. Is this useless extravagance, or a very effective service?

*DCh:* The questioner misunderstands PIs. All they are is a means of asking questions. So you put the question to the GP and he gives you an answer. I wish we could ask questions of the FPCs – there's a lot of very strange variations in general practice.

But, as others said in their turn, was any GP in a position to give a serious answer? If no one knew much about outcome in vast areas of medical care, just what was medical opinion worth? PIs certainly enabled questions to be asked. But were they the right ones and what did one make of the answers? Fundamental problems still remained.


## Nurse management information

Now consider another, equally crucial, difficulty. At first sight, the problems with nurse management information were much the same as those we have already described. There were, for a start, many key areas – such as the community services – where there was little or no information:

*UGM (community unit):* Well, the lunch was very nice but by the end of this morning's session I felt very guilty. Had I flattened the organization enough? And had I got enough vision? . . . I was going to describe my strategy – my management strategy, my financial strategy, my long-term strategy! And then a *problem* arose – called health visitors and things like that! (*loud laughter*) . . . The first thing that impressed me [when I started] was the amazing amount of competence and enthusiasm. But when I asked what people did, it was very hard to find out just what they did – in terms of precise output, outcome and so forth. And when I asked they all got very defensive – they didn't even tell me when I did a formal departmental review! [Speaker's emphasis]

*DGM:* We have very little planning in hand for the community services. The members have been very keen on developing these and getting more district nurses and health visitors. But there are no plans and no information on workload. The information that I get from the administrator in the community unit is that it's very difficult to get any information at all about nursing.

Moreover, even where nursing information systems did exist, the old problems remained – what did they actually measure? Workload measurement tools, such as Criteria for Care, tried to measure the nursing that patients needed and the care that nurses actually gave. Like clinical budgeting, the principles had first been developed in the United States and were now being applied here. And, although highly sophisticated, these too measured input, not output, process rather than outcome:

> *DGM:* You know Arthur's work [on Criteria for Care]. It's fascinating but it's really just – though at a much higher level – very fancy measures of input. I didn't know I'd done it but I rocked him right back on his feet when I asked why he'd chosen that particular point as the criterion for good care. It turned out that it was just because it was in the middle of the scattergram! There was no epidemiological input into it.

However, the most striking problem with nursing workload systems was not their absence of serious outcome measures, but their priority within the NHS. Those who defended clinical budgeting and performance indicators talked incessantly of the need to make a start, to begin somewhere. Doctors and districts were both crucial targets for evaluation. The new systems might have their problems but for many managers they were a big advance on what had happened before. With nursing, however, it was entirely different. Clinical budgeting was a priority for the entire NHS, so too were performance indicators, but systems such as Criteria for Care had no backing from the DHSS. Yet nursing was of central importance – and a massive cost – to the entire service:

> *CNA/Deputy DGM:* 50 per cent of our staff budget goes on nursing and it's 90 per cent of all direct care.

> *RCN representative:* The NHS functions more on nurses than it does on doctors. It's nurses who deliver most care and nurses who diagnose – you can't call it that but they do. Doctors rely on nurses' training – that they will call them when something's important and that they won't when it's not. Otherwise, doctors would have to be at the bedside 24 hours a day. So the system depends on nurses.

Such comments were more than mere professional self-promotion. In a heavily labour-intensive industry, nurses were by far the largest body of staff – half a million in all. As such, they also constituted the largest single component in NHS spending. Indeed, as a government report had shown, they accounted for nearly 3 per cent of *all public* expenditure.[2] Yet almost nothing was known about how this was spent and very little effort went in finding out. Thus, while some argued that there were far too few nurses to do the job, others insisted that there were far too many. No one really knew just what the huge nursing budget was used for or whether it could be used more effectively:

> *NHSBM:* A disproportionate amount of time has been put into areas of relatively low spending – for example, paramedics and pathology – and very little time has been put into nursing costs or other manpower costs which equal 45–50 per cent of the running costs of a DGH.

> *DFD:* There's a general feeling that nursing is under-resourced. This is true in some areas but not in others. We need careful studies to focus down on where this is true. We also need a recognition by the management group that resourcing at one level

produces a certain level of quality, while resourcing at another produces a different level. In the past, however, we merely resourced on an historical basis. We didn't know what the effect on quality of different levels of resource was – and we must know.

*CNA:* There's a considerable amount of fat in the budget. It's over-manned. Manpower estimates in nursing are at best unreliable and at worst an indictment.

*HSR:* I've also been producing information about the staffing ratios in mental hospitals. The range is threefold. Input doesn't guarantee output, but we do need to tackle the variations . . . The staffing ratios in many mental hospitals have been the same for many years – some possibly for a hundred years!

*DCh:* I'm quite sure that every district in the land has got problems here. My God, they [nurses] spout the jargon. If Jenny [nurse member on HA] would only cut this out, by God the content would increase considerably. She rattles on constantly about workload but she's no idea what she's talking about – and nor has anyone else.

*CNA:* We still haven't got the right information. We now know the numbers of nurses and the overall cost but what we haven't got is any estimate of how many nurses we need as the workload fluctuates. I make guesses, but we're strapped for answers other than professional judgement.

This last comment raises a central point. What was particularly worrying from a general management point of view was that the traditional method of allocating staff seemed as good as most of the more formal methods that had been developed over the last forty years. If medicine still rested on clinical judgement, the detailed distribution of the NHS's biggest resource was still largely a matter of the individual ward sister's unaided reckoning: of her experience, intuition and local, historical precedent. Consider the following exchange from a health authority meeting:

*CNA (presenting a report to a meeting of the health authority):* We [nursing advisory group] were very critical of the regional nursing manpower planning exercise. We firmly believe we need an increase. At The Royal [DGH] the nurses are really feeling the pressure. Staffing was fixed according to historical criteria but the throughput has gone on increasing . . . I'd like to pick up Mr Jones's [UGM] point about . . . tackling the overspend. If this is done at the expense of direct care, I'd be very worried. At The Royal, freezing posts has had a direct effect on us. There are no jobs for next week's group of finalists. The midwives have done a very detailed report on their workload in 85/86 and there's a real need for growth in midwifery manpower if the service is to be maintained . . .

*GP member on HA:* I was very pleased to see in the nursing advisory group report that it is necessary to find a formula for funding nursing manpower. I expect Jane [CNA] knows that this was discussed in the DMT from 1972 onwards and exactly the same things were said every year. Fourteen years later, we are still discussing exactly the same point as this every year – and it never happens. It's *got* to happen if action is to take place on nursing manpower. I was delighted to see it brought up, but unless some real action does happen here, nursing won't get the resources it wants. [Original emphasis]

*DGM:* Can I say that a number of formulae have been tried which haven't worked – that's been the problem.

Another CNA reflected ruefully on the failure of such formulae in a region in which she had previously worked:

CNA: I can remember when I was in the south-west, we used the Barr system [for allocating numbers of nurses to wards] and we ran that alongside a system . . . which relied entirely on the ward sisters' judgement. You couldn't have influenced the ward sisters, you had to take them whether they were newly in post and qualified for only two years, or whether they had fifteen, twenty years in post. We took off the top and the bottom and just smoothed it out a little bit and, having taken away these two extremes, what we were left with, I think, was about a difference of five whole-time equivalents out of a workforce of something like five hundred!

The new nursing information systems which were being introduced in some districts were a potential advance over systems like Barr and offered some possibility of more systematic management. However, unlike the other measurements that the new general management was forcing through at vast cost and at great speed, there was almost no action at all on the nursing front. Measures of performance were being introduced nationwide both for medicine and for district. There were no such plans for nursing. Systems, such as Criteria for Care, were a product of local, not national initiative and limited – on any serious scale – to a handful of districts.

Moreover, as the quotations below suggest, even in such districts, there were huge problems in sustaining the momentum. Vast sums of money were being poured by DHSS into those districts where the new approach to medical management was being readied. But nurse-management research was done on a shoestring and fitted badly with district politics and the many other demands that district made. All the quotations below come from the leaders in such research – not from the laggards:

CNA: The nursing budget in this district in £15 million a year, yet we spend just £15,000 on research.

DNS/NR: I was in a value for money post and when I saved half a million in the first few months the treasurer's department was very friendly – there were lots of shared committees! Relations began to go downhill as soon as the first results [from Criteria for Care] came out – and they got progressively worse when we said that no nurses should be made redundant as our staffing levels were inadequate for the new developments. On day one we were charming, on day five we were liars.

CNA: He [DGM] is a straight to the heart of things man, not an academic, but very bright. Unfortunately, he's inclined to see research as a frill activity.

NR: Jim [CNA] just heaps more and more work on me without a single thought about the resources that are needed to follow anything through properly. We can't go on like this. What's the point of doing bad research?

We have, therefore, a paradox. The development of routine systems for the effective allocation of nursing staff was of fundamental importance to both the cost and the quality of the NHS – and recognized as such by some general managers, treasurers, doctors and senior nurses, indeed, even by members of the NHS management board. But, when it came to the crunch, nursing was, once again, at the bottom of the heap. Nursing manpower was a huge long-term strategic issue, but when push came to shove, doctors were important and nurses were not.

Thus, for all the abuse that was heaped on the old nurse managers, it was far from clear that the new leaders had done any better. Although nursing might be vast and cost equally vast sums of money, nursing budgets were not there to be managed; or so it seemed to many nurses. Too many new managers thought simply of cuts and not of effectiveness. The weakness of the nursing unions and the rapid turnover of nursing staff made nursing an easy target; potential savings for any general manager in a little financial difficulty. Instead of facing up to the hard decisions and the massive long-term research investment that proper nurse management required, every hard-pressed district and unit had an easy way out:

CNA: I can't give details but in essence the new district strategy is to cease a large number of facilities – closing beds and saving on nursing salaries.

CNA: The UGMs are inclined to push the nursing needs to the bottom of the pile – 'Those nurses are always on about this' . . . Like saving £100,000 [on the new hospital]. 'Well, we needn't put in any new nurses.'

The problem was compounded by the way the service had been managed in the past. When nurses themselves had controlled the vast nursing budgets, relatively few nursing managers had shown much interest in systematic inquiry into the more effective use of nursing labour power. Such matters required a scientific skill, a quantitative grasp and a fundamental concern for modern management that was well beyond most CNOs. When most had thought of developing nursing, they thought, not so much of management, as of caring or of copying doctors, of the independent clinical professional and not the closely monitored labour force:

CNA: They [senior nurses] see it [nurse management research] so narrowly, not as a whole new way of life. . . As soon as you start to say how this will produce a real body of professional knowledge – if it's invested in – they start to turn off.

In short, throughout much of the NHS, nursing was trapped deep within a black hole. Those on the outside could not see in. Those on the inside could not see out. The largest and most expensive part of the NHS remained un-measured, unmonitored, ignored.

## Clinical advice, clinical quality?

Finally, consider one further vital problem with the new management's knowl-edge. The main information that a general manager needed concerned the product and the modes of production. The focus was, therefore, primarily on the clinical trades. The new leaders needed systematic data on the patients who passed through the service, on the treatments they received, on the myriad actions that doctors and nurses routinely performed. Such information was, however, embedded in two forms. It came not just in measurement systems but in people too. General managers needed advice from those with serious experience of the shopfloor – without it, the service would wither – or so many argued. Detailed measures of performance were crucial, but so too were specialists to interpret the new data systems, to liaise with the clinical trades, to spell out the science, the culture and the politics of the clinical worlds, both to create and to foster research. Specialist advisory staff were, moreover, essential, both to management and to those who worked on the frontline. Clinicians themselves were mostly focused on their own, individual work and, as such, were obliged to have a degree of faith in the efficacy of what they were doing. The perspectives of wider standards, of epidemiology, manpower, effectiveness and so forth were mostly alien to them without a good deal of understanding, encouragement and research.

However, just as there were major difficulties with the new systems, so there were also problems with these more personal tasks. Many of the old clinical managers had failed. Community physicians and nurse managers had often been too close to the clinical specialists and too inadequately trained in the skills of management. But now that they no longer managed the clinical trades, how far had the problem been merely reversed? General managers might know how to manage but, since they were generalists, how far did they lack serious operational understanding of the service and its needs? There was, so it seemed, still a very real need for the old clinical managers – or at least for their advice, if not their management skills. But, given the problems with their previous roles, could they do any better with the new tasks they had been allotted? There was, therefore, deep uncertainty over the role to be played by professional advisors.

In such circumstances, it is hardly surprising that there was considerable local variation, coupled with a general trend towards professional demotion. On the surface, doctors did better than nurses. After a short struggle with the BMA, the Secretary of State had insisted that every district must retain the post of DMO. By contrast, although every district was obliged to appoint a nursing advisor, in England at least, such posts did not have to be based at district level. But such relative triumph for the community physicians was often purely symbolic. In practice, DGMs could do much what they liked, whatever the formal structure. Though some DMOs were valued highly, many were not, and if nurse managers could be demoted, so too could community physicians:

> DGM: When I was at X district, I didn't like him [DGM of X district]. He's very determined and he was trying to destroy nursing. He didn't want a CNA. He's appointed a DNS as advisor and is now systematically knocking her off all the committees; mind, he's doing the same to the DMO.

Likewise, even where chief nurses were retained at regional or district level, some were still excluded from the inner workings of the district:

> CNA: I don't get a lot of the information now that I used to; the sort of thing that I used to get on DMT. I'm still on the executive team but now the DGM decides who on the executive team will see the correspondence.

*RNO:* I've not actually been excluded from anything. But the way it's happened, I'm just not told about things, I learn about them by accident afterwards. I'm not told I can't go. I just don't get to go.

*CNA:* I can choose what I offer advice on and I get to see all the papers beforehand, but I can only attend meetings which involve nursing policy and, obviously, one can't know just where the discussion will turn in advance just by looking at the papers.

Indeed, some new managers were so confident of their superiority that, at best, the old professionals' advice was ignored, at worst it was sneered at:

*CNA:* To him [UGM] I'm probably just another useless bureaucrat. When we were appointed, he turned to me and said, 'I'm going to be very busy. What the hell are you going to be doing?'

*DNS:* The UGM came to the old UMT meeting and it was really bad. He sat at one end of the table. The dialogue was exclusively between him and the administrator – and a little bit with the doctor. The UGM himself is an administrator. Everyone else was ignored. I was tremendously offended to hear someone else talking about my staff and not knowing the facts. I feel quite het up about it.

*DMO:* One of the UGMs is very nice and charming – and stubborn as a mule, i.e. he doesn't listen to my ideas! I worry about him listening to professional advice. He's very centralized. He wants to do everything himself – information gathering, planning, personnel.

There were many reasons for this major demotion of the old clinical management. Some new general managers desperately wanted specialist advice, but felt that the shortage of talent was so great that there was little possibility, as things currently stood, of obtaining anything useful:

*DGM:* The lack of a real DMO here is our biggest organizational weakness. I'm very worried about relations with the medical staff . . . The DMO is on the medical executive committee only as the lowest form of common courtesy.

Other general managers, however, may never have experienced good specialist advice and therefore did not know what they were missing. Yet others saw much of it as professional self-interest. In some districts, therefore, advice became merely an add on, an extra. Some specialists found themselves obliged simultaneously to offer professional advice to the authority, develop standards, and run units or other institutions – some of which were in a dreadful state and needed vast managerial input. How far real advice and serious quality could be developed under these circumstances was not clear:

*DMO:* There are districts like X where the DGM doesn't understand what community medicine does. The DMO has become a UGM as well. He gives the DGM advice but he's rushed off his feet. He can't do both.

*INT:* You say that you've exhausted yourself, your family, your energy.

*DNE/CNA:* Yes, I am drained . . . When the challenge came up, I felt enthusiastic. I felt that I could do a good job, that I could influence, could make nursing good in this district [both nurse education and nurse management had been in a terrible state when she had been appointed] . . . I welcomed it with both hands. But time is at a premium now . . . you feel, 'Oh, well, I can do it' and you stretch and stretch and stretch. I think one has to acknowledge that you can overdo it because you become ineffective after a while. You can do it up to a certain point and then it trails off.

*CNA/UGM/DDQ:* I'm between the devil and the deep blue sea.

So the new, hybrid roles could sometimes severely diminish the input from the specialists in clinical affairs. Much the same effect was achieved by demotion from district; or so many argued. In one-third of English districts, the new district nursing advisor was based not in the district management team but merely in one of its component parts – in the units. Yet units varied enormously. How far could advice on district-wide standards be given by specialists who were placed in a unit? And nursing constituted half the district's workforce and one-third of its revenue budget. Might it not be wiser for there to be someone at district level who could spell out the implications for nursing of district management's actions? Griffiths, after all, was about managing resources and nursing was the biggest resource of them all:

*CNA:* One person in one unit can't give unbiased advice to a district, because they only know about that unit. When I was DNS in X, I didn't give a damn about any other unit. I wanted as much resource as I could get for my unit. That's the name of the game. You need someone who can stand aside a bit; someone who can look at the district as a whole.

*CNA:* The situation in X district where I'm the nurse member of the HA is absurd. They've abolished the CNO's post, so advice to the district is given by a mental handicap DNS. He's a nice bloke, but it's a hopeless situation to be a mental handicap DNS giving advice to a teaching district. He just doesn't know anything on the acute side. It was daft, but as the nurse member I was being asked by the chairman to give nursing advice to the authority on things like major closure programmes due to their cash crisis! No one had pointed out that the closure of several wards which they had planned would have very severe effects upon nursing because these were also training wards.

In short, although there had been huge problems in the old clinical management, there were also great dangers with the new. Given the standards that seem previously to have existed among large numbers of community physicians and nurse managers, this may seem hardly a matter for criticism. If competent advisors were not readily available, there was little point in regretting the current downgrading. But according to some managers at least, there was still grave cause for concern. For them, the absence of a cadre of trained advisory staff was an organizational scandal of very considerable dimensions. Bridges did have to be built, operational knowledge was needed, native informants were essential and there was also a crucial role to be played in wider clinical research and development. Clinical quality was a very serious matter. And yet, so they feared, many new managers were quite unaware of the problem. Some of them, so it seemed, believed that they could run the service without serious professional advice; that a good suit, a little accountancy, a training in general management and a confident manner would provide all the answers:

*DMO:* It's OK here because Shirley [DGM] understands what community medicine does, but in some districts, DGMs just don't take advice. In X district, for example, the DGM is full of good intentions, but he's from industry, so he's completely ignorant about health care and totally in the treasurer's pocket. Treasurers don't like spending money – so everything is centred around this blinkered view.

*DMO:* The other thing that worries me very much is that we haven't set up the district in a way that will get good professional advice . . . Of course, some professional advice in the past was bloody awful – inward looking and self-seeking – but what's happening does worry me. We had a very good child health service here with a first-class SCM. The UGM is dismantling that bit and pulling it into a much less specialist form. We had thought hard about effectiveness and outcome – and I don't think the UGM knows what the words mean. If NHS management is going to be good, it's got to have good professional advice on outcomes. In a nutshell, this is what it's all about . . . We have a pattern of very devolved management in the community [unit] with managers from all kinds of disciplines. I want to know who'll set standards and quality at that level. I think that managers without professional knowledge of the end-point of the exercise will be very hard pressed. They may time-keep very well and look very smart in their nice pinstripe suits but will they know the questions to ask and the objectives to set? The old nurse managers didn't do very well but they did know some of the questions to ask. You would have to be a very smart general manager to know how to do this. I'm concerned about the lack of clarity as to what professional advice is. It's seen as an optional extra.

Of course, looked at from one angle, things might not necessarily be so bad. If advice was often problematic, there was, none the less, the beginnings of a major quality drive. In many districts a separate quality directorship had been created. On the face of things, all boded well. Yet some managers had serious doubts about this too. For a start, as we have already seen, for all the emphasis on new information systems, most data said very little about the quality of care. Cost was a priority; outcome was not. Such scepticism was reinforced by the way many districts appointed their quality directors. Many posts were given to the old DNO to be held as a hybrid with an advisory post. If managers appointed people whom they believed to be weak, how far were they seriously committed to quality? How far were such posts a form of outdoor relief for loyal but incompetent servants; or a way of appeasing region, the DHSS or the nursing profession itself for what had happened to nursing under Griffiths?

*DGM:* A lot of hybrid roles are just saying, 'We must find something for the poor old soul to do'. And that's not a good idea.

*DGM:* I could get professional advice from the unit nursing advisors, but I have to give John [CNA] a job, otherwise he'll be out of one. Not that I want to get rid of him. So that's why I've made him in charge of quality. Of course, the big problem is, what will the doctors say to a nurse talking to them about quality?

Not only might the introduction of quality directors introduce delicate political problems such as this, but creating real quality was an area of enormous technical complexity. Given the lack of investment in health service R and D, it was also an area whose research base was mostly lacking. Could the responsibility for service quality really be given to those who were busy on other things, who had no support staff, whose knowledge was focused on just one corner of the service, whose competence was in question or who had little or no education or research experience? And if such posts were created – but without any resources or active backing from the DGM – just what did that mean?

> *DMO/DDQ:* Some of the nurses in quality terrify me! . . . I've been really shocked by some of the ones I've met. They hadn't a clue. They thought it was all about dealing with patients' complaints . . . Some of the ones I've met think the idea is to get quality printed on T-shirts! . . . To give it to nurses just sets up the whole problem all over again.

> *CNA:* They're not looking at nursing standards [the district quality directorate], they've been looking at standards in the eyes of the consumer . . . I don't know how much the district is committed to [quality] in terms of funding. If you really want a standard nursing measurement you have to pay for it.

> *RGM:* If I'd been offered it [quality], I'd have turned it down. It's a minefield. There's no one thought about it seriously and because it's everyone's business, there's vast scope for conflict. And there's no resources specifically budgeted for it and a huge methodological war in the area. You can get very bogged down in it. If nurses try to pick it up and run with it, it could be disastrous for them.

> *CNA/DDQ:* It's ludicrous working on quality with just a secretary and a telephone.

How far, therefore, was much of the new emphasis on quality and the creation of quality directors simply a political gesture, a nod towards community medicine, towards patients, towards nursing – and towards the fashionable management writers of the day – but with little real meaning?

> *RCN representative:* I think the quality jobs are just a sop to consumerism. The managers aren't really interested in quality, just in efficiency . . . X now has the slogan, 'The Caring Region' – it's all just Saatchi and Saatchi [a well-known advertising agency].

> *CNA:* Industrial relations used to be the thing – that's how you got on in the NHS. Now the bandwagon is quality – that's how you get your picture in the papers!

## Conclusion

Griffiths was only a beginning. The new model created in 1984 was radical, but still a compromise with the very different tradition of central planning. Whereas writers such as Drucker had urged 'socialist competition' for this special type of service institution, the NHS remained a monolith. Griffiths might have installed a line of command and imposed a micro-management ethos but it had left the macro-structure intact. Besides, although Drucker had argued that in managing for performance, effectiveness, not efficiency was the key, many managers felt that the 1984 reorganization placed almost all its emphasis on cost – and very little upon quality. Huge attention was paid to finance, very little serious consideration was given to outcome. The long-term consequences of such bias were potentially dire; or so some critics argued. There was, therefore, still plenty of scope for reform.

# 12    1989 – towards socialist competition?

The Thatcher government never stood still. At the beginning of 1989, new proposals were made; the NHS was to be reorganized again. The White Paper[1] was sketchy and the negotiations were tough. At the time these words were written, the outcome was unclear and the government had yet to announce its actual legislation. But if the immediate shape of the new NHS was still unknown, the longer-term vision – and the strategy for reaching this utopia – was obvious enough. It is on this, therefore, that we shall concentrate in the rest of this account.

### NHS plc 1989 – the vision

Like 1948, the proposals were ingenious. Macro-principles on which the service had rested since its creation were to be abolished. Radically new alternatives would take their place. That abolition would, however, be piecemeal. The new system was to be created just a bit at a time, as individual institutions 'opted out' of the old organization. No comprehensive new structure would be formed at one stroke of a minister's pen. In the new vision, the NHS would be freed from direct interference by politicians and civil servants, floating off from Whitehall as a quasi-independent corporation – NHS plc at last. That corporation, however, would be very different from the old. The NHS had provided services for defined populations and did so on a largely monopolistic basis. There was little competition between GPs and none at all between hospitals. Now, however, doctors would start to compete for patients as well as resources, while DGHs would have to compete with one another and not just the local community unit. In the process, or so it was hoped, they would be forced to jack up their standards; the market would apply its own sanctions to all those who failed.

The method was simple. Just as the service would escape from the clutches of politicians, so units would be set free from the close grasp of district. Indeed, districts would eventually disappear, save for a small rump that would be merged with the local family practitioner committees that had supervised general practice. Each hospital would become a self-governing entity, free to compete both on cost and on quality with every other hospital; free to hire staff and pay wages in the way that it wanted. The new market for NHS health care would, however, take a rather special form. Real competition needs clients who can choose. Yet almost all patients were massively ignorant of bio-medicine and many of them, by virtue of their very status as clients, were weak, disabled or seriously ill. Doctors, inevitably, tended to dominate the relation-ship. The new vision had three answers to this age-old problem. Like the 'socialist competition' to which Drucker had referred, the NHS market would be regulated from above. The role of the NHS board and of regions would no longer be to plan and to integrate services but to monitor and regulate standards – and to do this not just for the old NHS units but for the private sector too if it wished to join in. (Provided it agreed to regulation by NHS plc, any hospital could become a medical supplier to the service.)

In the new method of control, regulation was the key. Regions would monitor standards through new performance indicators backed up, at long last, by enormous investment. A huge growth of management R and D would ensure that the quality of the service was maintained. So too would a new type of health authority member. The amateurs of the past drawn from many local interests would be replaced by men and women from professional management, people who already knew how to make organizations perform and could cast a cold eye over their colleagues in health care.

Finally, since patients were often in no position to choose, doctor would be set upon doctor. The firm British division between the hospital consultant and the general practitioner would be put to yet another use. GPs had long con-trolled hospital referral; now they would buy in the hospital care for their patients, choosing between hospitals to get the best deal that they could. They, in their turn, would be tightly controlled. Their deals with the hospitals would be monitored, their services would be advertised (they also would now com-pete with one another) and they would, for the very first time, get a budget. The financial discipline of cash limits would extend throughout the whole service; and so too would a systematic monitoring of medical care. A new, sharp-eyed service would be born, both more cost-effective and more con-sumer oriented, ready for the major demands of tomorrow – for the inexorable growth of technology, for the rising burden of the elderly.

In 1984 only nurses protested. In 1989 almost everyone did. But this was a government not prone to pay much attention to protest. Like a good many radicals, Mrs Thatcher believed that the British people were deeply alienated from their own long-term interests. It was the job of government not to listen and consult but to instruct and attract – to command a new order, to train people in its ways and to pay keen attention to that immediate self-interest which, so she held, motivated much of human life. So the orders went out to that single line of command, that chain of general managers from the top to the bottom of the service whose new, short-term contracts made them eager to obey. The machinery for fundamental restructuring was already in place. And if some managers were upset, others were already thinking that way. Just as some districts had begun Griffiths-style measures in the years immediately before 1983, so the same was true of 1989. Consider these extracts that were recorded three years earlier, each in a different district:

*DGM:* I've mixed feelings about the regional tier. It hasn't moved quickly enough to separate the general management function from the services it provides. It only needs twenty people for the general management side. Everything else could be put on a profit centre basis and simply charged to districts – though we are moving a bit in that direction.

*CNA/DDQ:* I think that very shortly the ward sisters here will buy in services from the catering department – this is getting near the stage of completion . . . and the units buy in my department's services. For example, the other day, a unit administrator came in and said could he have four weeks of Chris's [DR] time to look at secretarial support. Joan's [DDR] time is also bought in by the units. We charge £25 an hour to any of the units who want the services of my staff. Our aim is to be self-sufficient. The private nursing homes buy in their staff education from us too. The units do have a choice. The alternative is to buy in the services of Price Waterhouse or someone like that – which is far more expensive . . . My aim is to produce a quality of care within the NHS which people will buy from us rather than buying in X [local private hospital]. We've also got three work study engineers and they too sell their services to the units . . . I really like the idea of building things like saunas and selling them to the public! The board meets next Wednesday to discuss this. We've already got a privately let cafeteria.

*DFD:* 'Contracting district services' – Jim [DCh] gave me a clipping from the paper about this and I've had a brief chat on the phone with this chap in X district. He said he had tried to refer cases to Y district via the GPs but the GPs weren't cooperating. He said they were under enormous pressure from region – as they were RAWP-gainers – to do something about their enormous waiting lists. So what they're trying to do is buy a ward.

*DGM:* And do Y district also get cross-boundary allocation and get paid double?

*DCh:* All the more reason for doing it!

*DGM:* Brian [RGM] says this is illegal and I always thought it was right outside the NHS.

*DCh:* I think Brian may be out of date on this . . . It's just like a district contracting with a private hospital.

*DFD:* I said to him that I thought we were one of the most cost-efficient districts in the country.

*DED:* Should we advertise our services?

*DFD:* How about a letter to the RGM of Z [the region in which X district was located]? . . .

*DGM:* As for X district, I think we should go ahead on that one.

*DFD:* Should we write to all the HAs and look to see who's got very long waiting lists?

*DCh:* This is what PIs are for. Write to those with long waiting lists in the RAWP-gaining areas.

Here, then, was the new kind of service in embryo, keen to cut costs and push quality, convinced that a new form of competition was the way to do both. What can be made of such claims? The question is important, not simply because health care is vital, but because the latest reforms are merely one instance of a new mode of government which has swept right across the public sector; a mode which is no longer just the property of Mrs Thatcher's administration but has stimulated interest in almost all shades of political opinion. Yet in health care, general management is a doctrine whose effects are still largely unknown, while some of those who have introduced it have been massively doctrinaire. Some radical right traditions have an interest in empirical evidence others, like some of their counterparts on the left, argue solely from first principles.[2]

In consequence, although many aspects of general management may offer real and important advances in the control and distribution of health care, there is plenty of scope for things to go wrong. Its techniques can be applied in many different ways and, since the old NHS had some remarkable virtues – whatever its other failings – a good deal of caution may sometimes be called for. Thus, just as we began with a chorus of criticism for the old NHS, so now we conclude with some sceptical reflections on the attempts to apply modern business management to health care.

### The new dilemmas

Take first the character of the new order of things. General management is both a theory and a practical discipline. As a theory, it is not something that has been conclusively and scientifically demonstrated to be superior; nor, perhaps, could it ever be for it operates in that most complex of worlds, the social arena, the home of the soft, not the hard sciences. Thus the only way practical managers can proceed is by using a subtle brew of hard evidence and gut feeling, of official statistics and qualitative data, of both careful analysis and the charismatic enthusiasm of management gurus, variously stirred. General management, in short, is a philosophy, a paradigm, a doctrine. These difficulties are increased, in public services at least, by the sheer novelty of what is now being attempted. Socialist competition is a hybrid whose qualities – although potentially attractive – are as yet empirically unknown. There are no old hands to talk to, no maps or well-worn guides to follow, merely theoretical blueprints. The ideas are interesting – but do they work?

One thing, at least, is certain; there will be vices as well as virtues. If social science lacks the precision of physics or chemistry, some propositions still get a measure of general assent. One such concerns the fundamental role of un-intended consequences in human affairs – a proposition that is as central to Adam Smith as it is to Max Weber or Karl Marx. Health seems no exception to the rule. Just as the old NHS had its downside, so an NHS plc may expect a few problems of its very own making.

One sort of issue concerns the essentially local nature of most health services. With its emphasis on integrating the trades within a service, on flexible forms of local administrative structure and on the systematic monitoring of individual performance, general management does pay very close attention to this feature.

But, there are other local aspects, at least in its fully competitive form, in which it may, perhaps, do rather less well than the system which has existed up till now. Those aspects concern access, equity, local representation and the integration of one service with another.

The start up costs for entry into the hospital market are extraordinarily high and most parts of the country – with the exception of just a handful of very big cities – have only one hospital of each type. Real competition between hospitals would, therefore, involve a huge increase in the distances which patients have to travel. Yet ease of geographical access seems to be a fundamental wish of most health care consumers. In consequence, there may well be either a very large number of dissatisfied patients and relatives, or alternatively, local hospitals may still end up as monopoly suppliers of most local services.

Geographical equity, too, may be a problem. Forty years of struggle and planning have created, by most international standards, a fairly high quality service in almost every part of the country. (Inner City general practice is, perhaps, the one great exception.) Can a system which comprises competitive units do as well? RAWP and its equivalents are being abandoned and the hope now is that the market combined with national regulation will continue to force up standards and do so more effectively than the previous system. But competition is prone to many imperfections and markets can often produce great inequities in distribution. The situation will need very careful management.

And what of local representation? Health services affect us all and community representation is just as essential as professional expertise; indeed, both are needed. Too many of the old health authority members may have been ignorant and amateurish, but is this sufficient excuse to sweep away the whole notion of representation of all sectors of the local community? Finally, a key aim of the 1974 reorganization was to integrate all the health and the social services in a particular local area. Such integration is fundamental to those common conditions in which the services of many different trades and institutions are required – physical handicap is a classic example of the problem. Competition between hospitals may possibly make sense for cold surgery – for cholecystectomy, for example – but how much relevance does it have for those many other conditions where patients need a whole range of services and need them urgently or on the spot?

A second area of concern is that of cost. This too has been a key focus for general management action, yet will the model now being unveiled really control costs? Might it not, instead, actually increase them? Again, there must be serious worries on this score. The old NHS was extraordinarily cheap, as the American managers of Johns Hopkins had admitted when addressing their colleagues in Britain:

USGM: The world over, forces are aimed at limiting admissions and cutting the cost of health care . . . I know we spend 11 per cent of GNP to your 6 per cent. I know we have 4.4 beds per thousand and you have 2.2 – our planners are trying to get to

2.5. I know we have 2.2 consultants per thousand and you have 0.3 – we're trying to get to 1.5 . . . We're not here to talk about that to you (*pause*) the experts in resource limitation (*laughter*), we're here to talk to you about management style. [Speaker's emphasis]

The new NHS management style was largely borrowed from the United States – but would it fare any better than it had so far done in its country of origin? In one sense, the question is unfair. American health managers start from a very different level of provision and work within a very different system from the one currently being planned in Britain. There has been no American equivalent either to the NHS or to NHS plc. There are nevertheless some grounds for suspecting that the new system proposed here might add to, rather than cut overall costs.

One major reason for the economy of the old NHS was the abolition of the fee for service principle. Since individual items of care were not charged for, the vast bureaucratic expense of assessing that cost was avoided. But in NHS plc, fee for service is central to the whole operation. If services are to compete in the provision of care, each item must be carefully priced. There are other costs too. Individual monitoring of the quality of care is extraordinarily expensive. So too is the abolition of collective bargaining. Dealing with a million individual employees involves vast investment in management training, time and systems.

And what of the costs to the clinical staff? Doctors have been trained at enormous expense to be specialists in medicine. How cost-effective is it if they are all to become mini-managers and if all of them now need to spend time negotiating patient care deals? There are also costs to the patient. Choosing health care is a complex, often delusory business, yet most talk of the virtues of markets assumes that choice is pure benefit, cost-free. In fact, most evidence suggests that what patients want is a convenient, local service, not the huge burdens of choice and long-distance travel. Finally, how far will real competition actually be possible – and if it is not, just how efficient will the system really be? Not only may many local hospitals remain monopoly suppliers, but there are other serious constraints upon competition. If hospitals and GPs are not allowed to drop unprofitable lines, how efficient can they actually become? Competition often depends upon specialization. Different producers concentrate on what they do best. But if the regulatory apparatus insists that each supplier offers a reasonably full array of services, what, then, is the consequence for the overall cost of the system?

Quality is a third major problem. As Drucker repeatedly says, all organizations need efficiency but above all they need effectiveness – a fundamental emphasis on the right results. Yet, as Chapter 11 revealed, although many new managers talked about quality, there must be grave doubts about how much they actually know about the subject. Since this is so, what happens to all the bold claims that are made for the new order? How can the vast new regulatory structures work, if there are few indicators of quality? How can managers direct the work of individual doctors in any rational fashion if they are ignorant of most medical outcomes? Some advances may certainly be made on the basis of the knowledge we already have – but can a whole health care system be erected on this basis? In economic theory, the benefits of competition are premised on the assumption that purchasers possess serious information about the product. But, in health care, both parties – producers and patients – are all too often profoundly ignorant. And since what information there is rests almost solely in medical hands, can managers really seize power from the profession – or are they still doomed to bow to traditional medical might?

There are other problems. The old claim that health care is different rests, not just on the absence of technical information, but on, so it is argued, its unusual moral properties. All social life is suffused with morality but in health care, which deals with suffering and the very preconditions for life, moral questions take a particularly acute form. One obvious point concerns the value of life. Actuaries, generals, judges and economists can – if asked – all put a practical cost to a life but few, if any, outsiders see them as possessing much insight into how we ought to estimate its real worth. Indeed, the democratic, humanistic and religious moralities that inform both our public and private lives all typically insist that the matter is incalculable. Health care, not surprisingly, is profoundly influenced by these arguments. In our study, some of the most fervent exponents of general management still felt that health care was a special case, set apart from the business world and deserving somewhat different treatment. The first speaker below had joined the NHS from private industry; the second was a tough ex-administrator:

DGM: The first question we have to ask is, what is the product? Our previous speaker [a well-known businessman] has helped me along these lines. So what is the product? Health care. It comes in three forms – preventive, curative, palliative. Of course, it changes all the time. The NHS is what's known commercially as a jobbing shop. But our product is health care – if we recognize this, we have a common objective . . . [But] what is the difference between a commercial organization and the NHS? If a commercial organization is to succeed, its members have to identify with it. If it fails it's because, perhaps, their contribution to it is wrong. In managing commercial organizations everyone moves in the same direction – except in moments of madness. But in the NHS, all kinds of forces make this impossible. It's very difficult to have just one objective. [For example] a professional dealing with a patient has a one to one relationship which transcends organizational concerns. Take the case of George Hammond – that policeman who was slashed so badly – doctors threw budgets out of the window. It's the same with nurses too . . . [Likewise in the NHS] there's a personal and emotional side. We have to deal with patients who are frightened and worried. This puts huge pressure on us; far greater than the pressure customers put on Burton's.

DGM: I find the whole concept of Qalys quite frightening. [Qalys were a proposed method for assessing the value of patients' lives, the effectiveness of different treatments and the resources which should therefore be given those with particular conditions.] Logically, I can agree with it, but morally I find it quite frightening. Public sector management should have only two cheers for effectiveness. It needs to fudge that last little bit.

The unusually intense moral nature of health care, its inescapable links to duty and to each individual, cause other problems too. How much is the fellow feeling that tribalism produces a moral bonus and not just a weakness? Might individual assessment and individually fixed pay destroy teamwork, rather than help integration? Might competition turn clinicians into salesmen and sales-women, with fixed smiles like airline cabin staff? And what happens to the cleaners on short-term contracts? How far might they now become, not a part of the team – however lowly – but a grudging, resentful, wholly rather than partially exploited servant class? In short, is the ethic of competitive, monitored performance actually quite what we want from a health service? Might soli-darity and collectivity still be important principles of organization?

Finally, what of the interests of the rulers themselves? General management makes much of the vices of specialists, of their tribal, self-interested qualities. So what, one may ask, are the vices of managers? Not surprisingly they turn out to be just like the others, for general managers are specialists too. Expert in management, fascinated by cost, but ignorant of outcome and mostly unaware of quality, how far may general managers come to focus solely on the things they know best, on the parochial issues that concern their own tribe?

## Conclusion

For a conclusion, we go back to the beginning of this book. One hundred and fifty years have passed since George Whistler introduced general management to the Western Railroad of Boston. Yet in health care, at least, the vision still seems a very long way off. A single line of command can be created and, so too, can decentralized management but real competition and continuous perform-ance assessment are much more difficult to achieve. Real markets are hard to create in health care. Patients want a local and immediate service, while hospi-tals come in multi-million pound lumps, not in packets like soap powder, and are, therefore, very few and far between. And, while real competition depends on generally available information, well-informed participants – whether patients, doctors, nurses or managers – are in very short supply. Though every-one wants better outcomes, who knows how to measure them? And just what is the role of local managers in health care when most serious data on the performance of their institutions are lacking?

These are difficult questions, but health care has always presented intractable problems. The new model of management, the new vision of markets, may both offer – with one great proviso – major tools for its better organization. The proviso is this: the new methods of managing for performance are fine – just as long as the new managers' performance is also rigorously monitored. The experiment needs careful analysis.

So far, however, the government has shown little interest in such assessment. The evidence that clinical budgeting has largely failed to work has been ignored. Proposals that the new system be tried on an experimental basis in one region have been set aside. But perhaps assessment cannot be expected immediately. Democratic politics is driven by elections – and we are all politicians of a sort. There is no long-term incentive for actors to take part in truly radical experiments when a new government might set everything aside. In the United States major formal experiments in health care organization have, indeed, taken place. New systems have been tried out and evaluated in experiments which have cost millions of dollars and many years to complete. They rest, however, on a very different footing to any found in the UK – on a belief in social science that Great Britain does not share and on a much greater consensus between the political parties.

All that may change. The Thatcher governments' aim – throughout the whole society and not just in health care – has been to abolish the old forms of consensus management and create new forms of consensus based around markets. Such radical change requires great faith – and leaves little room or time for debate and systematic evidence. Research takes many years, but breaking an old agreement and establishing a new one requires rapid and decisive action.

Insofar as Thatcher has succeeded in creating a new British consensus, formal experiments may become easier in the future. Market socialism can be operated by the Right and the Left and there will be much to experiment with. The 1989 reorganization will, no doubt, still be a major compromise with the past. Change will inevitably be slow. Doctors have still to be controlled, nurses have still to be noticed. Many areas will prove hard to bend to the new model. Health care, in some respects, will always prove an exception – but much about that exception is still to be discovered. Shrewd guesses can be made, but there is always scope for human ingenuity and innovation, as well as for great error. We must hope that our managers are wise as well as bold.

# References

## Epigraph

1. G. Rosen, quoted in R. Guest, 'The role of the doctor in institutional management', in B. Georgopoulos (ed.), *Organizational Research on Health Management*, Institute for Social Research, University of Michigan, MI, 1972, p. 289.
2. R. Burns, On the late Captain Grose's peregrinations through Scotland, 1789.

## Foreword

1. K. Hoskin, 'Boys from the blackboard', *The Times Higher Educational Supplement*, 24 March 1989, p. 14.
2. P. Strong and J. Robinson, *New Model Management: Griffiths and the NHS*, Nursing Policy Studies 3, Nursing Policy Studies Centre, University of Warwick, 1988.
3. Department of Health, *Working for Patients*, HMSO, London, 1989.
4. D. Cox, 'Health Service Management – a Sociological View or, Griffiths and the Non-Negotiated Order of the Hospital', in M. Bury, M. Calnan and J. Gabe (eds), *The Sociology of the Health Service*, Routledge and Kegan Paul, London (1990).

## Chapter 1

1. Department of Health and Social Security, *NHS Management Inquiry* (The Griffiths Report), DA(83)38, DHSS, London, 1983; Department of Health and Social Security, *Health Service Management: Implementation of the NHS Management Inquiry Report*, HC(84)13, DHSS, London, 1984.
2. P. Ross, quoted in B. Deer and T. Rayment, 'NHS team set for purge on doctors' perks', *Sunday Times*, 17 March 1985.
3. J. Robinson and P. Strong, *Professional Nursing Advice After Griffiths: An Interim Report*, Nursing Policy Studies 1, Nursing Policy Studies Centre, University of Warwick, 1987; J. Robinson, P. Strong and R. Elkan, *Griffiths and the Nurses: A National Survey of CNAs*, Nursing Policy Studies 4, Nursing Policy Studies Centre, University of Warwick, 1989.
4. B. Glaser, 'The constant comparative method of qualitative analysis', *Social*

*Problems*, 12, pp. 436–45, 1964; P. Strong, *The Ceremonial Order of the Clinic*, Routledge and Kegan Paul, London, 1979.

5. P. Strong and R. Dingwall, 'Official discourse and the limits of action in formal organizations', in P. Abel and N. Gilbert (eds), *Accounts in Action*, Gower, Farnborough, 1983.

6. G. J. McCall and J. L. Simmons (eds), *Participant Observation: A Text and Reader*, Addison-Wesley, Reading, MA, 1969; M. Hammersley and P. Atkinson, *Ethnography: Principles in Practice*, Tavistock, London, 1983.

7. J. Roth, *Timetables*, Bobbs-Merrill, Indianapolis, IN, 1963.

8. E. Goffman, *Asylums*, Anchor, New York, 1961.

## Chapter 2

1. A. McGuire, J. Henderson and G. Mooney, *The Economics of Health Care; an Introductory Text*, Routledge and Kegan Paul, London, 1988.

2. A. Hirschman, *Exit, Voice and Loyalty*, Harvard University Press, Cambridge, MA, 1970.

3. P. D. Fox, 'Managing health resources: English style', in G. McLachlan (ed.), *By Guess Or By What? Information Without Design in the NHS*, Oxford University Press for Nuffield Provincial Hospitals Trust, Oxford, 1978, p. 10.

4. R. Klein, *The Politics of the National Health Service*, Longman, London, 1983.

5. Ministry of Health, Scottish Home and Health Department, *Report of the Committee on Senior Nursing Staff Structure* (Salmon Report), HMSO, London, 1966; Department of Health and Social Security, *Management Arrangements for the Reorganized NHS* (Grey Book), HMSO, London, 1972.

6. DHSS, *Management Arrangements*.

7. R. Hutt, *Chief Officer Career Profiles: A Study of Backgrounds, Training and Career Experience of Regional and District Nursing Officers*, Institute of Manpower Studies, Brighton, 1985.

8. H. Glennester, P. Owens and A. Kimberley, *The Nursing Management Function After Griffiths in the North-West Thames Region: Interim Report*, London School of Economics, London, 1986, p. 5.

9. K. Middlemas, *Politics in Industrial Society*, Andre Deutsch, London, 1979; C. Barnett, *The Audit of War*, Macmillan, London, 1986.

10. Quoted in P. Hennessey, *Whitehall*, Secker and Warburg, London, 1989, p. 590.

11. *Ibid*.

12. Department of Health and Social Security, *NHS Management Inquiry* (The Griffiths Report), DA(83)38, DHSS, London, 1983, p. 12.

13. Department of Health and Social Security, *Health Service Management: Implementation of the NHS Management Inquiry Report*, HC(84)13, DHSS, London, 1984.

14. P. Drucker, *Management*, Pan, London, 1979, p. 20.

## Chapter 3

1. See J. P. Martin, *Hospitals in Trouble*, Basil Blackwell, Oxford, 1984.

2. R. Dingwall, A.-M. Rafferty and C. Webster, *An Introduction to the History of Nursing*, Routledge and Kegan Paul, London, 1988.

3. J. Robinson, P. Strong and R. Elkan, *Griffiths and the Nurses: A National Survey of*

*CNAs*, Nursing Policy Studies 4, Nursing Policy Studies Centre, University of Warwick, 1989.

## Chapter 6

1. T. J. Peters and R. H. Waterman Jr., *In Search of Excellence: Lessons From America's Best-Run Companies*, Harper and Row, New York, 1982.

## Chapter 7

1. P. Salmon, 'Cures and curiosities', *THS*, December 1985, p. 5.

## Chapter 10

1. C. Webster, *The Health Services Since the War*, Volume I, HMSO, London, 1988, p. 2.
2. P. Drucker, *Management*, Pan, London, 1979, pp. 154, 155 and 158.

## Chapter 11

1. P. Drucker, *Management*, Pan, London, 1979, p. 158.
2. National Audit Office, Report by the Comptroller and Auditor General, *National Health Service: Control of Nursing Manpower*, HMSO, London, 1985.

## Chapter 12

1. Department of Health, *Working for Patients*, HMSO, London, 1989.
2. P. Dunleavey and B. O'Leary, *Theories of the State: The Politics of Liberal Democracy*, Macmillan, London, 1987.

# Index